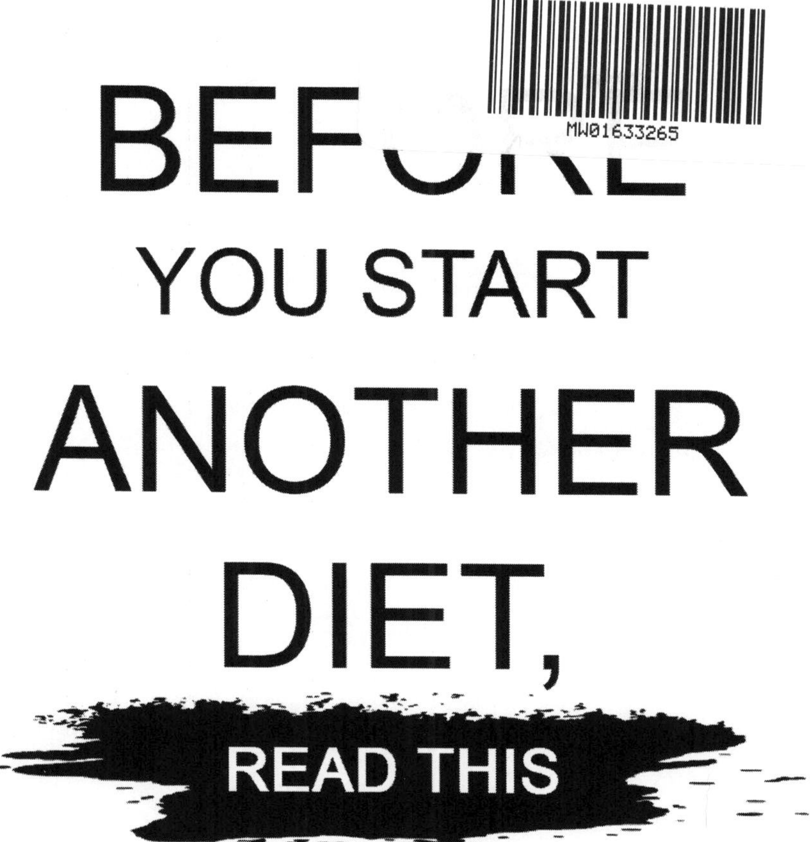

BEFORE YOU START ANOTHER DIET, READ THIS

Unsubscribe from the Diet Culture, by Focusing on the Inner Work of Self-care

RHONDA ARMOUR

The authors of this book do not dispense medical advice or prescribe the use of any technique as a form of treatment for physical, emotional, or medical problems without the advice of a physician, either directly or indirectly. The intent of the authors is only to offer information of a general nature to help you in your quest for emotional and spiritual well-being. In the event you use any of the information in this book for yourself, which is your constitutional right, the author and the publisher assume no responsibility for your actions.

The views and opinions expressed are those of the authors. Although the author and publisher have made every effort to make sure all information is correct at press time, the author and publisher do not assume and hereby disclaim any liability to any party for any loss, damage, disruption caused by stories with this book whether such information is a result of errors or emission, accident, slander or other cause.

Paperback ISBN: 978-1-7386873-3-6
Hardcover ISBN: 978-1-7386873-2-9
Digital ISBN: 978-1-7386873-1-2

Table of Contents

Chapter 1

The Journey Within

Do you ever wish someone could climb inside your mind in order to understand your thoughts and the conversations you have with yourself? And if they could experience your thoughts and feelings, it would become clear as to why you struggle and why you have started then stopped so many diets or self-care programs in the past? Why you just can't accept your body the way it is and why you have so many insecurities?

It can be a lonely place. A frustrating place. That place inside your head that is always searching for the answer, for the right way, for that one thing that will click and finally work.

The societal pressure to look a certain way is immense. The assumption that in order to be successful or worthy, we need to be a certain size, weight or shape somehow defines how we value ourselves. By seeking this external validation we are limiting our ability to see ourselves for who we really are and what we are capable of - all of which have nothing to do with what we look like on the outside.

Then we turn around and look to those same external influences for answers on how to take better care of ourselves and how to feel better about ourselves. Is it the latest diet that all the Hollywood stars are on? Is it a personal trainer? Yoga? Therapy? Is it the newest smoothie diet to hit social media? The list goes on. Yet we never stop to consider what role we, ourselves, actually play in managing our thoughts and actions relating to our body, nutrition, physical activity, and our overall self-care. We don't stop to consider that perhaps the answers and insight can be found from within.

It can be scary to do that, I suppose, because then we would have to be honest with ourselves. We would have to really dig deep to understand what causes us to make the decisions we do and what holds us back from being able to appreciate and love ourselves. It would require us to be vulnerable and admit that we have a much bigger challenge on our hands. We would need to engage in the process of managing our minds and every thought we have tried so hard to run away from so that we don't have to face ourselves.

It's so much easier to give someone else or some random program the reins and put them in the driver's seat because then we are released of the responsibility should things fall apart. We don't have to do the hard work. We can simply follow the program's instructions and rules, and we are suddenly absolved from dealing with what's going on within our own minds. That doesn't work for long though, as we continually start and stop new programs with little to no success in changing what we look like or how we feel about ourselves. Instead of seeing the program for what it is, an unsustainable, unhealthy and unrealistic approach, we start to internalize the lack of success and it becomes yet another thing we have failed at. It's our fault. We are now a failure and all blame can lay heavily on us until it's time to find another "solution" to put our hopes and dreams into. And the cycle continues.

There's absolutely nothing wrong with wanting to lose weight or wanting to be a different shape or size. You can want that for yourself for a variety of personal reasons and still not get there. Or you could get there and still not be content. You still may not like what you see on the outside because you haven't done anything to change the inside. Inside your mind is where the change needs to happen. This isn't about how much weight you want or think you need to lose, what society deems is an acceptable size or shape, or anyone else's opinion about your body. This is about you being healthy physically, mentally and emotionally. This is about acceptance of your body and looking at making changes, not because you hate what you see, but because you want to love what you see and want to feel amazing inside and out.

I know plenty of individuals who accept their bodies, no matter their size. They love themselves and their bodies, and I'm thrilled for them and the self-acceptance and freedom they've developed. Being healthy isn't about a number on the scale or being a specific size, and it certainly isn't a gauge as to whether you should feel confident and comfortable in your own body. That's a personal feeling that you get to own. Every woman deserves to be happy and healthy in her own body, and the only opinion that really matters is her own.

The reality though, is there are many women out there that are concerned about how they look, always searching for ways to be healthier and never happy with how they look and feel. They're lost and unsure if it's even possible to feel comfortable in their own skin again. It pains me to know that women are struggling because I know that pain all too well. Admittedly, I still struggle with that pain; certainly not every day, but often enough to know that it's not an enjoyable way to live.

There may be past trauma or current emotional and mental health issues that can impede us and hold us back from making progress. There could be obstacles and limiting beliefs that aren't easy to overcome, or perhaps can't be overcome at all. I understand that for each individual, there are reasons for the way they see themselves and the way they feel about themselves. There are likely deeper issues at play and I admit, this is beyond my scope. I can only speak to what I have struggled with and what work I've done to make small mindset changes that have helped me get to a better place. A place where I understand what I'm capable of and how my mind works, a place where I know I deserve more than how I've treated myself in the past.

Remember, this is not about the number on the scale, the size you wear or who has more weight to lose; it's about how you feel about your own body. I've struggled internally with body image, with my relationship with food and with the fear of gaining weight for as long as I can remember. The feelings still live within me, but my approach to seeing past them is very different now.

I'll tell you though, if I could turn back time, I wish I had the ability to recognize and understand that I own the rights to how I take care of myself and how I value myself. That I could trust myself and didn't need to rely on others to create standards or expectations for how I should look or feel. It could have eliminated years of struggling with my weight or at least the thoughts I had around my weight. I could have developed a better relationship with food and would have been able to take better care of myself, mentally and physically. Perhaps even being able to love and trust myself enough to engage in thoughts and actions that would have allowed me to be free of self-judgment.

My drive to support those around me comes from a place within that has worked tirelessly to block out the voices that tell me things I know in my mind aren't healthy, but in my heart, (or maybe it's the vain side of me) things I can't get past. That voice that holds me back from loving myself fully, on the inside and outside. It takes work to dispel it and to understand that just because the voice came from within me, *it doesn't represent all of me.* This will always be a work in progress and I'm okay with that.

I'll be honest. I'm not famous, I'm not skinny, I have depression, I don't have a million followers on Instagram, and I live in a little town in Ontario, Canada surrounded by farms. But I do have concepts and experiences that I believe will provide you with a starting point to better understand yourself and explain why other programs out there haven't worked for you. In my opinion, you haven't been taking the right approach and have been misled, time and time again, by diets and programs that are designed to fail in order to keep you coming back. You've stepped away from all that you know to be true because you have not developed a firm sense of who you are and what you are capable of doing. You have been misinformed and it has changed what you say to yourself, and about yourself.

Within my coaching business, I absolutely advise clients on nutrition, exercise, and all things self-care, but to be honest, we spend so much more time talking about the psychology of weight loss, body image, what their internal dialogue looks like and what is really holding them back. I'm by no means a therapist and don't claim to have all the answers, but I can ask the questions so we can attempt to get to the root of the struggle. It's fascinating that we, for the most part, know what to do in order to be healthy, yet we don't always do it. That is what I want to explore. What it is that holds us back and how to proceed in a way that is constructive and meaningful. In a way that doesn't involve you having to follow a diet or program that wasn't made for you. I'm hoping to enhance your understanding of yourself as you move through this book, and have you explore and examine your thoughts through a different lens so you can start taking steps toward self-acceptance and the freedom to embrace *custom* self-care.

Again, this is the starting point of your journey. There may be deeper healing that needs to be done based on your personal experiences and story, but my hope is to lay a foundation for you. The barometer for success in this book is not weight loss though. It's the *inner work*. Although, I have to admit that, for me, my focus back then was always strictly weight loss. This has changed for me over the course of my own journey as I learned to take into account who I am as an individual and create strategic habits that worked for me. Throughout this book, I want to share my own stories and experiences with you, so you can understand the perspective I'm coming from, perhaps even be able to relate to things I had done, thought or felt in those times. I want you to know that I hear you and I get you. I want to speak about what I was taught within the diet culture or what I believed I needed to do in order to have confidence within my own body. This will be about my own healing, as much as it is about sharing my knowledge around creating a healthy lifestyle for yourself.

I want you to understand that you're not alone because chances are, I have felt, thought, done or said the same things you have. I crave genuine well-being for myself and I want that for you too. This will look different for every one of you out there. You are on your own journey. The helpful habits I will speak about are ones I found to be helpful and ones my clients have found to be helpful as well. I want there to be a new definition of success and new solutions when it comes to the help that is offered to those of you struggling with body image and feeling uncomfortable in your own skin, whether you want to lose weight or not. This is just the beginning, a jumping-off point where we will focus on the tools to help you get started on your journey.

I want to have you consider different strategies and concepts that I classify to be the inner work. The foundational pieces that act as the leg work I believe you must dive into before moving forward with changes to your self-care lifestyle. Looking at whether you are ready, willing and able to move forward in your journey is an important topic we will explore, along with creating custom strategies that are unique to you. We will dive into various perspectives around the concepts of trial and error, determining your why, making small incremental changes, setting yourself up for success, establishing your non-negotiables, saying no and setting boundaries. We will do a deep dive into the importance of choices and how choice can create empowerment. Part of the inner work will include the importance of creating a support system, understanding the role of discipline versus motivation, and being consistent rather than perfect. Finally, we will discuss unsubscribing to the diet mentality which I know might feel daunting. We want to break the cycle and recognize that you deserve more than what diets have to offer.

Please understand that you don't need to start implementing all of the strategies and habits all at once. In fact, it's better if you don't. *One habit at a time, one day at a time.*

There has to be another way and there has to be a different dialogue that's present in society. I also strongly long for there to be a different dialogue that takes place inside your own mind. I know that the steps I've taken in the past, physically and mentally, to feel better about my body haven't always been healthy and I'm not sure, to be honest if I will ever be able to entirely step away from my focus being on weight loss. Yes, I'm focused on being healthy and yes, I love to be strong and yes, I love to be an amazing example for my kids and clients. At the end of the day, I'm doing what I can to change my thoughts because those are what have kept me in this place of self-doubt, being so tied to weight loss and so tied to the fear of gaining weight.

It is my commitment to continue to change, grow and learn, and I'm extremely passionate about having it be different for you too. In fact, when I spoke to my publisher and those that have helped me along the way to get this book up and running, I cried. Probably for two reasons: one, because it brought up so many wounds I have kept deep inside about my own struggles and my unhealthy mindset when it comes to weight. And two, because it breaks my heart to think that other women, like you, are going through what I have and feel you are the only ones when, in fact, you are not alone.

This is real.

We're not just talking about health, being a particular size or shape, or any other vanity ideals. We're talking about being able to love yourself again. I know that might sound cliché, but isn't that what you really yearn for? To be honest, even now I can't imagine truly loving how I look on the outside, but writing this book and impacting the lives of other women is part of my healing process and I want to infuse that into this book. I'm hoping to empower you to do the same for yourself so you can perhaps change the path you're on before you get too far down it. Only you know how you feel about yourself and only you know when you are truly taking care of your entire self in order to be the best version of you. At the end of the day, you need to be able to love and trust yourself to know that you are doing the best you can for your mind and body.

We need to talk about this. About how you want to feel about yourself, your desire to love yourself both inside and out, and the disconnect between that and your actions. It's not talked about enough. Unfortunately, I never had anyone to talk to me about my struggles in the past and it forced me to take on this incredible internal burden that no one should have to endure. You have to stop this overwhelming desire for a quick fix or this thinking that someone or something can fix how it is you feel about yourself. Whether it's a diet, a fitness program, a gimmick to drink shakes for weight loss, or any other program; *you deserve more than what these programs have to offer - ways to shrink your body. And nothing else.*

I want to talk about the big picture. And the big picture requires the inner work. How you take care of your physical, mental and emotional health. It matters, and it's taken me a very, very long time to recognize that, so I'm hoping we can have a real conversation that might spark something in even just one person. That one person just might be you.

If you picked up this book thinking it would lead you to yet another diet or self-care program that promises you weight loss or some other form of body image success, you grabbed the wrong book. And if you're honest with yourself, you know you don't want another one of those books. You're tired of those books. You know the books I'm talking about. The cookie-cutter ones that you know are impossible to follow but you try anyway because you are desperate and if it's in a book, it must work. The thing is, those books aren't *made for YOU*. The you that has a career, kids, relationships, obligations, mental health concerns, responsibilities, and so much more.

BUT if you picked up this book because you've had enough of fad diets and programs that have left you feeling lost and empty inside and are finally looking for real change, stay right here. It's not a magic formula, though. It's about getting real and calling it like it is—an honest discussion about the internal work required to take better care of yourself and change how you think about yourself.

I want you to feel amazing in your body and proud of what it's capable of, regardless of your shape or size. In order to get there, steps need to be taken so you can confidently know that you are taking an active approach to mental and physical well-being. This is not like all the books out there telling you how to eat better, exercise more effectively, or lose weight, all while not knowing the first thing about you, your lifestyle or how you feel about yourself. There can't be a one-size-fits-all approach. There's no logic behind that when you are all unique individuals with your own stories. So before you consider moving ahead with yet another diet, read on and consider a fresh approach.

Chapter 2

I Am Human Too

I want you to understand that I'm a real person, just like you. Working in the industry I do, oftentimes others will assume that maintaining a certain appearance or fitness level comes easy to me. *It doesn't.* I've had various obstacles and experiences that have shaped who I am and how I operate. I think it's important to paint a picture for you outlining a little about my history before we dive into the concepts and habits I want to share with you throughout this book.

As far back as I can remember, I have struggled with depression and, if I'm putting it all out on the table, I'll admit that I can probably count on one hand the number of people in my life that know this. This is not because I'm ashamed, it's just one of those things I've kept close to my heart. As a child, I always had this overwhelming feeling that I needed to cry, even when I wasn't sad. It was the strangest thing, so my mom started recording these occurrences on a calendar so we could show my doctor. No real diagnosis came from it, but it was recommended that I seek out a psychologist as it was likely a mental health issue versus a physical one. I have absolutely no recollection of my time in therapy or if it did anything for me. I guess eventually I just stopped going, but as I got older, the concerns around my mental health became even more prevalent.

Through my early 20s I was struggling quite a bit and things really came to a head after the birth of my first child in 2005. Postpartum depression hit me like nothing I'd ever experienced before. It was pretty immediate, starting at the hospital, where I felt no connection to my baby girl. Once we got back home, all I did was cry. I felt such huge regret for what had just taken place in my life; I didn't want this child. This wasn't what I signed up for and I had no interest in being a mom. It was like I was having an out-of-body experience as I couldn't recognize who I had become and didn't understand the thoughts I was having. I wasn't allowed to be left alone for fear of what I might do, and I had convinced myself that I would never get through to the other side of what I was feeling. This was my new reality and the blame was placed squarely on my baby girl. I wouldn't have wished this experience on my worst enemy.

I remember a day when my sister came over and offered to take my daughter for a walk. I so badly wished she would just keep walking and never come back. That would be the answer to everything. I believed I would be better off if I didn't have to take care of this child.

What sort of state must I have been in to have such a thought?

The first few months of being a new mom are a blur. I'm not quite sure how I was taking care of a newborn when all I remember doing was crying and trying to claw my way out of this deep emotional hole I had fallen into. To make matters worse, I was struggling to breastfeed, but the guilt of even thinking about giving that up was just too much to bear. This just compounded the darkness I felt and this feeling of overwhelm was constantly present. Thankfully, with the help of my husband, mom and family doctor, I received medical attention and was put on an antidepressant to help balance my hormones. The following few weeks were still very much touch and go as I had to allow time for the medication to take effect. During that time, it was literally a day-by-day process of healing and understanding what was happening within. I almost had to get reacquainted with myself and the new life that was upon me. Having thoughts you know are not really yours and ones you aren't in control of can take its toll on how you view yourself.

Gradually becoming more aligned with who I really was as a woman and a new mom was certainly a period of difficult transition. Over time, the person I always knew myself to be started to re-emerge and I was able to recognize myself again. I embraced being a mom and finally got to experience the love for my daughter I had missed out on in the beginning. It still amazes me to this day how quickly things spiraled for me after giving birth and the impact unbalanced hormones can have on your mental state. Then on the flip side, the dramatic impact the right medication can have to turn things back around. There's a sense of how fragile we really are when you reflect back on the experience, having come full circle.

I eventually came off the antidepressant but still knew that something wasn't completely right. The depression tendencies were still present, but at the time it really wasn't being talked about and I wasn't sure what to do with my feelings. So I kept plugging away at life. I knew I wanted another child, but the thought of experiencing postpartum depression again was daunting. I had worked so hard to get to a place where the love for my daughter was at the center of my universe. I couldn't wrap my head around how I could possibly have any more love to give to another child. A friend at the time explained to me that I didn't have to divide my love and instead, I could multiply it. That gave me the peace I needed, and a few years later, I had my second daughter. This time I was prepared and had my antidepressants on hand, just in case. Once again, I found myself in a place all too familiar, but at least those around me saw what was happening so we were able to take a more proactive approach.

My oldest daughter is now 17 years old and depression has been present in my life up until today. Between therapy, practicing self-care, surrounding myself with people that get who I really am and medication, I'm able to move forward. It's always there though. I've tried to come off of the medication a couple of times, thinking I would be fine without it, but it doesn't go well. The hormone imbalance is just too great for me to handle. So I've accepted the fact that antidepressants are likely a part of my forever, but so too are other measures, such as staying active, eating nutritious food, getting enough sleep and effectively managing my stress. It all plays a role in my physical and mental health.

As you can imagine, it would be much easier for me to negate my self-care and give into the depression. But it's just not in my personality, and my kids deserve better. I'm a solution-oriented person so I'm always having to make adjustments to ensure I'm where I need to be in order to be at my best. That being said, I'm not always at my best. Internal and external factors play a role in that, but I refuse to accept that just because things are the way they are, they need to stay that way. No. We have to think outside the box.

A factor that likely plays a significant role in my mental health is the chronic back pain I live with on a daily basis. I have scoliosis, which means I have a curved spine. As a result, I have degenerative discs and all sorts of other alignment issues that cause other issues throughout my body. The pain doesn't go away – ever. It's always there in varying degrees and, to a certain extent, I have learned to live with it. Some days are good and some are unbearable. I've been through extensive care from acupuncture to physiotherapy to massage therapy. I've seen an orthopedic surgeon that said my back wasn't bad enough "yet", that eventually my discomfort would go away because the discs would be so worn down that it wouldn't cause any more pain.

This meant the pain would eventually be substituted for limited mobility, according to what he told me. Needless to say, the guy was an asshole and I never went back. I refuse to believe what he said, so I do what I need to do to take care of my back. As you can imagine, there's a direct link between my chronic pain and my depression. Those that suffer from chronic pain often also suffer with mental health concerns such as depression. There's a part of my brain that has to focus daily on managing the pain. At certain times of the year it can consume my mental capacity and can bring me to my breaking point. I'm still bound and determined to get my 5-7km walk in every day though, and do some weights to keep my strength up. It's both physical and mental therapy for me.

As I reflect back on my childhood, I can't ever remember having active conversations around healthy nutrition, positive body image, or self-care in general. I apologize to my parents if this happened and I just don't remember!

The thing I do remember is always struggling with poor self-image and confidence regarding my body. I always hated my body and there was never anything close to experiencing body positivity. I've always avoided looking in full-length mirrors and I can't stand having my picture taken. I've always been super sporty though, playing rep baseball. At school I got into volleyball, basketball, lacrosse and even did track and field. I still brag to my kids about winning the female athlete of the year award in school which, as you can imagine, they aren't always thrilled to hear about. I also won the French award back then, but I'm less inclined to brag about that particular one…If you asked me to right now, I couldn't even speak it to save my life! Anyway, back to the topic at hand, I likely got lucky that I was able to maintain my weight growing up due to my involvement in sports, but once those activities slowed down, the weight started to creep up. Unfortunately, weight has a tendency to go up if you don't engage in regular exercise.

Regardless of where I was on the scale or what I looked like, I never felt good in my own skin.

I always had an unconscious relationship with food and used food to cope with a variety of emotions, which is actually very common. I used it as a coping mechanism when things weren't going my way. Whether it was being unhappy in my career, struggling in my marriage, going through issues with friendships, or having that constant feeling of not understanding where I belonged or what my purpose was, I tended to utilize food as a way to feel better. I wanted to ignore those nagging feelings of being unsuccessful or unimportant. I suppose back then, food was the one thing I could at least control.

Over the course of my adult life, I had engaged in so many diets and programs that most of the people in my life had no idea about. Trying to navigate the rules and restrictions of those programs during holidays, celebrations and social gatherings was challenging because there's a sense of shame that follows you. You feel like you need to hide what you're doing from everyone for fear of judgment, I suppose. Most people in my life understand that I am very conscientious about how I eat, getting my exercise in and all of the other self-care habits I engage in, but they had no idea the impact it was having on my mental state or the lengths I was willing to go in order to change what I looked like on the outside. It's not something I was proud of because I knew deep down I was taking the wrong approach.

The control it had over me is quite remarkable. It used to be all I thought about. When I got to eat next, what I was going to eat, and how excited I would get about food. On the flip side, I was always seeking out a new fad diet. I participated in programs like Weight Watchers, Dr. Bernstein, Atkins, and other various diets I'd seen on television, took pills that promised weight loss, and went through hypnosis and countless other measures just to be thin. You can only imagine the role this played on my mental health as I was desperate to find a solution. Desperate to experience self-confidence and feel positive about my own body. This went on year after year, even while I was actively pursuing my personal training certification.

I'm sharing all of this with you not to create a pity party, but to help you recognize that we all have things going on inside and in the background of our lives that might not be evident to those around us. Whether it's physical or mental, there will always be challenges and obstacles in your life that may slow you down, but remember that these challenges and obstacles should not limit your ability to move forward.

I, too, have real problems, baggage from my past, and things that slow me down, so perhaps you see a little bit of yourself in me. The struggle is real, as they say. Whoever "they" are; and it's hard. I will never pretend it's easy because I would be lying. Shame on those in the diet industry and those on social media that simply tell you "do this and do that" and portray an ease about making changes to your health. There's nothing easy about it. It frustrates me that while they are quick to dictate the rules and regulations of their diet or program, they are also quick to hide from the real issues that people are dealing with, capitalizing off of how you feel about your own body. They know you're unhappy with yourself and are selling the hope of *feeling* better by *looking* better. There's never anything included about the mindset issues you are dealing with because it's solely about weight loss and becoming smaller. They are in no position to give advice or impose rules when they know nothing about you or your story.

I always find it interesting how people think they know me or draw conclusions based on what they see on the outside. I've received comments about the fact that I always have my hair and makeup done, I'm so dedicated to my power walking, I'm present on social media with such a positive attitude, I have a successful coaching business, and so that equates to me having it all together. Behind the scenes, you never know what people are dealing with and what challenges they are facing. I'm human and still struggle from time to time, and I'm honest with my clients about that. I don't paint this perfect picture and create a false sense of security around how easy the process of taking good care of yourself is, day in and day out. My day-to-day method is to listen to myself. To trust myself. To pay attention to the dialogue I'm having with myself and to remain present.

I often struggle with imposter syndrome, which is defined as "an internal experience of believing that you are not as competent as others perceive you to be." I have to continuously remind myself that just because I struggle with my own body image and my relationship with food from time to time, it doesn't mean I can't help other women. In fact, I think it can often be an advantage to truly understand what they are going through. There's a relatability factor there and I'm actually listening and hearing what my clients are saying and going through.

I'm looking to adjust the perspective you have of yourself, but I know you have to want it and that I can't simply want it *for* you. I care so deeply about other women like you and the challenges you face when it comes to how you feel *about* your body and *in* your body. I see myself in you and don't want you to struggle unnecessarily, and especially not alone. I did that for far too long. I have always been a perfectionist and extremely hard on myself, and I know it's not helpful in moving forward. I don't want you to be so hard on yourself; I want you to understand that you are better off showing yourself kindness and grace for real change to transpire.

I recognize that after many years of chronic dieting and unrealistic expectations of myself, it's not helpful to live solely inside our own minds, going round and round looking for solutions and being critical of ourselves. I encourage you to open your mind and allow me to be your cheerleader, while being a realist, and my hope is that during our journey together through this book, *you can become your own cheerleader.*

24

Chapter 3

Making It Personal

For some reason, as women, we are not great at making it all about us. It's about the kids, significant others, our careers, family, friends, and a million other things. I think that's because it's so much easier to take care of everyone and everything else than it is to really do the hard work of taking care of ourselves. It's also a societal expectation, if we're being honest.

We've all heard that if you don't have your health, nothing else really matters, but for some reason that still doesn't seem to resonate with us. Is it because we think we have time to figure it out down the road? Is it because we truly believe that all of the other things in our lives are more important than our health? Is it because we think the world would fall apart if we didn't take care of everyone and everything else first? I don't know the answer, but something is holding us back and we need to get to the bottom of it. Or should I say, *you* need to get to the bottom of it. I completely understand that self-care is often a matter of privilege and not everyone has a partner or the means to make it a priority. So within your means, I encourage you to think about the reasons you have *not* made your self-care a priority. A *consistent* priority.

I once had a fascinating conversation with a client who is a successful business owner, and she told me that as she was getting her business up and running, there were many times she got knocked down but still continued to get back up and push through. She stressed that failure was never, and is still never, an option for her. At that moment, I commended her drive towards the creation and growth of her business and asked why there were limitations on the dedication and commitment she had to her self-care, but not to her business? How was the success of her business any different than the success of her self-care? I asked with no judgment but as a powerful analogy, and it stopped us both in our tracks. It was a fantastic moment that had our wheels spinning and there was no solid answer that could be provided.

We do this, don't we? We put so much energy into everything else, but not ourselves. It's the easy thing to do, I suppose.

But I believe that you deserve better. The question is: Do YOU believe that you deserve better? Do you ACTUALLY believe it? If you don't ACTUALLY believe it, then nothing will change. I want you to take your power back. The power you have over your own thoughts and the power you have over the decisions and choices you make. You have the power whether you recognize it or not, and it's time to reclaim it, stand in it and believe in it. The process of undertaking new self-care habits doesn't start with you simply making changes like exercising more, eating healthier meals, going to bed earlier, or drinking more water. You can't just dive right in, it won't last. It starts with taking your power back. You have to do the pre-work. The self-reflection. The inner work. You have to answer the tough questions. Often the tough questions will stop you in your tracks.

Questions like:

    Are you READY?

    Are you WILLING?

    Are you ABLE?

But you need to be honest.

If I were to be honest about where my level of "readiness, willingness and ableness" was to take on a healthy approach (mentally and physically) to losing weight in the past, I now know I was missing all three pieces right from the beginning. Starting back in my early twenties, I had an incomplete understanding of what it actually meant to be ready, willing and able, and I carried this misinformation with me for many, many years. If I had taken a real look at where I was mentally and emotionally with regard to my body image, I would have known that I had some serious work to do. All I knew or cared about was instant weight loss results, and I wasn't willing to hear anything that would get in the way of me achieving those results.

I certainly wasn't ready to accept that I had emotional issues that were strongly intertwined with food. I was definitely not willing to address those issues and, in the beginning and for many years after that, I wasn't able to even understand that this was a problem that had a very big impact on my ability to keep weight off. The only problem I could see was the fact that I had weight to lose. I couldn't see beyond that. Of course, if a diet didn't work or if I couldn't stick with it, it had everything to do with those beliefs, and no consideration was given to the limitations of the diet itself.

We can say all day long that we are *ready* to do what it takes to maintain better self-care, we are *willing* to take action to improve our self-care, and we are *able* to do what it takes to get where we want to be. In the end, I feel strongly that we aren't seeing the big picture. We aren't ready, willing and able to dig deep enough within ourselves to recognize what it is that truly holds us back. We're engaged in surface thinking. We only consider the specific actions and behaviours that are apparently required of us to feel better about ourselves. Actions such as putting healthy food in our body, exercising, getting enough sleep, drinking ample water, meditating, journaling, and so on. Anyone can follow a diet, a workout program, a meditation course or anything else that someone else has designed and you simply follow. What determines if you have created sustainable habits that allow you to feel positive about yourself, is whether you have done the inner work. That has to come first. This is where I fell short for so many years. I simplified it in my mind that if I just did X, Y, and Z that my latest diet dictated, it would equal the results I so badly craved. This would then equal increased self-confidence and a positive image of my body. Well, the equation just isn't that simple, and never will be no matter how hard we try to manipulate it.

Are you **ready** to do what is required for change to take place?

Are you **willing** to do what is required for change to take place?

Are you **able** to do what is required for change to take place?

Again, you need to be honest. Answering these questions is part of the inner work. It doesn't serve you to pretend. You're only setting yourself up for failure. *You want this time to be different.* You want it to stick this time. You are in it for the long haul.

Sometimes your answer will be NO and that's ok. Doesn't mean it's going to be NO forever. Just not right now. Better to wait until you're READY, WILLING and ABLE than to make a false start, or several.

If you've answered YES, and it's an honest YES, I want you to realize that the process of undertaking new self-care habits has to be all about *you* and getting to the place where you have acceptance of your body. Understanding your 'why' is the key, as well as understanding what it is in your life that will be made better if you were to make these changes and reach your goals.

This can't be about you doing it for other people or for vain reasons. There has to be a bigger picture. I want you to think about how you will *feel* and how you will be different on the *inside* if you reach success, and what your definition of success really is.

I encourage you to raise the bar and the expectations you have of yourself. It's time to step up to the plate and crush that ball (for those of you that don't know me, I'm a huge Toronto Blue Jays fan so excuse the baseball analogy)! It's important to hold yourself and your actions to a higher standard. If you have goals around losing weight, building muscle, increasing your energy or just feeling awesome about yourself, I encourage you to expect a little bit more from yourself, each and every day.

When it comes right down to it, you have to ask yourself if you are ready, willing and able to do the hard work and circle back to whether you believe you are deserving of the hard work and the results that go along with it.

This is where the custom strategies and solutions come into play. The process of how you move forward to reach your goals has to be all about you. What has worked for your friend, sister, or co-worker, doesn't necessarily mean it's going to work for you. If you haven't done this inner work to determine what will actually work for *you*, it will likely just be yet another "thing" you have tried. The fundamentals of good health are the same for everyone. We need to eat nutritious food, move our bodies, get good quality sleep, manage our stress, stay hydrated and focus on our mental health. The difference in how we manage to be successful in these areas is based on you as a person. It's based on *your* lifestyle. There is no one-size-fits-all approach.

For example, there has to be a custom strategy for how you will change your nutrition and start eating healthy meals and snacks. It's not good enough to just say you're going to start eating healthier. What does that even mean? How are you going to manage that with your busy lifestyle? How will you ensure you can maintain these healthy eating habits? It's certainly possible and we can all do it, but the implementation process has to consider how you live, day by day, what sort of mindset you have and what changes you can see yourself sticking with long term.

It's not good enough to just say that you're going to start managing your stress better so you can help keep your hormones balanced and avoid stress eating. What does that mean for you? How are you going to do that? You need a custom game plan and the plan has to factor in your mindset and the stressors you have in your life.

When developing your custom strategy, I want you to consider things such as:

Your work schedule

The school hours and extracurricular schedules of your kids

Your significant other's schedule

Your most productive and energetic times of the day

Personal and professional obligations

Community commitments

Previous strategies attempted

Seasonal weather changes

Personal interests and hobbies

Physical and mental health limitations

Anything else that could impact you achieving your health goals

Not only do you have to consider the logistics of your life, you have to also be realistic about your mental capacity to embrace and implement the changes you're looking to make, and that's where it can be challenging. We often overlook this part or just assume we'll be able to handle it. I don't want you to assume, especially if you know you've struggled in the past. Instead, I want you to recognize that you are not doing yourself any favours to overextend and go beyond your capacity. Be confident enough to recognize when you are getting close to your personal mental capacity, and slow down or dial back accordingly.

This process is not easy and this is coming from someone who does this for a living. I struggle too. You have to see the big picture, and the big picture includes your mental health, your emotions, who you are as a person, the stories you tell yourself, your past experiences, and your current lifestyle. Each of us has a story based on many years of ups and downs, programs we've tried, gimmicks we've bought into out of desperation, and it's time to rewrite the story one sentence at a time, and this time, the ending is different and final.

I want to paint a picture for you that explains how distorted my thoughts were when it came to my weight and body image. I'm not going to pretend that these thoughts still don't creep up and impact my actions and behaviours, because they do, but I'm happy to say that it's not nearly to the same degree as it once was.

As far back as I can remember, food has been a focal point in my life. There were constant thoughts about food. Looking back, I recognize that it was an obsession. An obsession with food. It dominated my thoughts. I would live for "cheat" days and would literally count down the days until I got to overindulge in foods that I thought would bring me great joy. There was this constant awareness of how I was feeling in my own skin and it was never positive. I always felt uncomfortable, thought I was fat, and was hyper-aware of every single flaw. I was constantly thinking about how much weight I had to lose or what I had to do next in order to lose the weight because I was so scared of being overweight. There wasn't a day that went by that I wasn't engaged in these thoughts and this overwhelming desire to look different. To look better. I avoided looking in mirrors or having my picture taken because I couldn't stand the thought of seeing what I thought I looked like. My whole self-worth was dictated by my weight, the number on the scale, the size of my clothes and how I felt in my body. These thoughts were always there, day in and day out. My self-worth was never linked to my personality, to what I had to offer the world, to the impact I was having on others or to my ability to perform at work or as a mom and wife. It *never* crossed my mind even once before.

I'm glad to report that that is no longer the case. I've surrounded myself with wonderful people that make me realize I am more than just my weight, and with that, I had to do a lot of internal work to find what self-care habits work for me. What habits keep me feeling mentally and physically healthy, what habits I know I can maintain long-term and what habits fit into my lifestyle. I do have to admit that the view of my external being is still a work in progress and likely always will be. I'm ok with that. I've grown to understand what would be involved for me to achieve the look I *believe* I want, and I know it wouldn't be good for my mental health if I were to take that on. The habits and structure just wouldn't fit into my lifestyle and I've had to be realistic about what I'm *ready, willing* and *able* to do. There's a balance that I have to strike and that's where the daily inner work comes in.

I want you to recognize that you need to start doing this for yourself, not for those in your life. Others will have opinions on what works and what doesn't, and how you should proceed with taking better care of your health. Oftentimes other people don't recognize that just because *they* think you look great, you might not think that way. The opinion of others doesn't suddenly change the way you think or feel about yourself. *That has to come from within.*

At the end of the day, they don't know what will work for you. They don't know how you're feeling or what you're thinking about yourself, no matter how well they know you. Only you know. In my experience working with clients, it quickly becomes apparent that their friends and family aren't always on board with the changes they are trying to make. This usually comes out of the guilt they're experiencing when they see you trying to take better care of yourself. This is when they push food on you, tell you to skip the gym or have one more drink with them. We've all experienced this. This makes them feel better about their crappy choices and in your effort to avoid conflict, you end up compromising your own success and giving up on the commitments you made to yourself. In fact, you may have found yourself being that person trying to sway others away from their healthy habits just to make yourself feel better. It's not right, but it seems to be human nature.

I have a client that had come to realize that her choices around alcohol were really impacting her ability to make good food choices, as well as her energy levels and her ability to lose the weight she so badly wanted gone. A big part of her life was the social aspect of gathering with friends, partying and weekend getaways where alcohol was always present and consumed; oftentimes, in excess. This was no longer working for her so she made the decision to stop drinking for a couple of months in order to stay focused on the goals she had committed to. As a result, other people started questioning her decision, disrespecting it as they pushed alcohol on her, even going as far as ridiculing her by claiming she didn't want to have fun. These reactions caused my client to be angry with how she was being treated, and disappointed that the people in her life weren't able to get behind her and be supportive of the choices she was making. It felt like high school all over again where she was experiencing peer pressure to do something she wasn't comfortable doing, except now she was a grown-ass woman!

She was not making this decision lightly and it was not done to please other people. Her goal was to take better care of her health and feel better about herself. Had she had an illness where she was unable to consume alcohol she would have received all the support in the world, yet when she decided to take a step back from it in order to feel better, she received flak for it. We had many discussions around the reasons why other people act in this way and about standing firm in her decision. Once you can see other people's intentions, it's much easier to feel confident in the decisions you are making for yourself.

Other people will constantly try to influence and shape your decisions, whether it's consciously or not, maliciously or not. Again, this is where we circle back to whether you ACTUALLY believe you deserve better from yourself. If you believe, you will be able to stand strong in your beliefs and the commitments you have made to yourself, and simply decline whatever it is others are offering or trying to push on you. Again, it's hard. It takes practice. Over and over again. This is about you and your health and it's time to get selfish. We've all heard the saying that self-care is not selfish, and it's not. If you don't take care of your physical and mental health, who will? The responsibility rests with you, and the sooner you can wrap your head around that, the more effective you will be in reaching your goals. You have to stop looking for programs and people to solve a problem only you, yourself, can solve. You can rely on resources for education and talk with experts to get questions answered, but at the end of the day, it's on you. *I want you to own it.* Empower yourself and become a leader in the quest for good health and feeling amazing about your body.

So, what is your *why?*

It sounds so cliché, but you have to ask yourself. We can't keep playing the victim of diet culture because it will always be there. Trust me, I played the victim for a very long time when I would try a new diet, fail, and then have difficulty understanding why it didn't work or why I didn't magically feel great about my body. I thought it was unfair that I had to work so hard just to lose weight. I wasn't being honest with myself though. It wasn't even about the weight. It was about my *thoughts* relating to my weight and my body. I was looking for the easy way out and wasn't willing to look inwards. Instead, I was searching for someone or something to make it easy. You have to start getting real with yourself about *why* you want to look better and feel better. If you know why, you'll be better equipped to take on the work that is required to get there.

It's disappointing to think that for so many years my "why" was to be thin. To look good. Pure vanity. It had nothing to do with my health, my kids, being the best I could be, my energy levels, aging well, or any other solid reason. That's the truth. I understand that the desire to look good isn't something to be ashamed of, but I also understand that it can't be the sole reason to engage in self-care habits. It's not enough. There isn't enough on the line. I'd never considered my "why" because I was so hung up on losing the weight and assuming that once the scale went down, everything else I was feeling about myself and my body would magically fix itself. I never stopped to consider that if I were to lose the weight and become the size or shape I envisioned in my mind, I still might have these lingering issues to face. Well, that became evident when time after time I did, in fact, reach my weight loss goals yet I was still left yearning for more. Not more weight loss, but more in terms of how I felt about myself. I still felt uncomfortable in my own body. I still doubted whether I could keep the weight off. I lived in fear that if I gave up the ridiculous diets, it would all slip away.

When I looked in the mirror, I still saw the excess weight or the problem areas and was continuously overanalyzing what it was I was seeing. I wanted to be proud of how I looked and wanted to finally feel good living in my own skin, but these were only fleeting thoughts. The fact that I hadn't gotten real with myself about my "why" is what allowed for the vicious cycle to continue. Even after losing weight I would gain it back, only to then look for another way to lose it. I can now see that one of the reasons for that was because I hadn't actually addressed the underlying issues and hadn't done the inner work. I had no understanding or had ever given any thought to my "why" and the role it played in holding me back.

I have had many clients that were once yo-yo dieters and when I ask them to explain why they stopped each diet even when they had success in losing weight, it causes them to pause. Why would you stop something that worked? They would normally go on to talk about how the weight loss wasn't worth the sacrifice and they didn't feel they were being nourished.

They just couldn't live like that long term. Or they would comment about how difficult it was during gatherings or vacations and once they stopped it was too difficult to start back up again. The fact that they had lost weight didn't seem to matter enough to stick with the diet. Although they had success and changed the way their physical body looked, they hadn't changed their mindset or thoughts about their body and hadn't uncovered what it was they truly valued. We know they didn't value being told what to eat or measuring and weighing everything they ate. They didn't value having foods that were off limits, a bunch of food rules to keep track of or being hungry all the time.

What we did establish is that they wanted knowledge, choices, control, a plan, energy and the ability to feel strong and healthy. Rarely do they actually say they want to lose weight! That normally ends up being a bi-product of the work they do and the understanding they gain about taking care of themselves in a healthy way. So I encourage you to find your why or at least start to consider other reasons for you to take better care of yourself. Do your homework, self-reflect and understand that there has to be more to it than losing weight and being smaller. There has got to be something more important to you than simply wanting to weigh less, and that can then become your driving force. That is part of the inner work.

Consider answering these questions:

How do you want to feel mentally about how you take care of yourself?

How do you want to feel *in* your body and *about* your body?

How are those you love impacted by you ignoring your self-care?

How do you want to feel as you age?

What does your health hold you back from experiencing?

How would your life be different if you took better care of your health?

Be specific and detailed. Nobody else has to see your answers. You are trying to get to your deeper why and uncover what it is you truly value, so honesty is the best policy here.

I've admitted that stepping away from weight loss being my primary focus has been difficult, but with time and a better understanding of myself, I can now confidently say that my why is linked to my health, both physically and mentally. I now know that I need to eat nutritious foods, move my body, get enough sleep, and engage in all of the other self-care habits, so I can continue to live my life full of energy and feel my best. So that I can travel, hike amongst nature, create memories with friends and family, be there for my kids and their kids, and can continue feeling strong in my own body. Not just so that I can be thin. That was never a good enough reason.

Chapter 4

Trusting the Process

As I've previously said, this is hard stuff. The solutions for taking charge of your health and changing the way you think about yourself are not easy. You're looking at ways to take on self-care habits that will allow you to feel confident in what you are doing and allow you to remember why these self-care habits are important to you.

TRIAL & ERROR

At times it can be a little bit of trial and error, which you might think is absurd, but in my experience coaching clients, it's the truth. Because you're looking at custom strategies and solutions to integrate healthy habits into your world and change the mindset you have around those habits, sometimes you have to try a few things out before they stick or before you can wrap your head around them. As the saying goes, "third time's the charm". Or fourth or fifth or sixth. It has to work for you otherwise it will constantly feel as if you're trying to fit a square peg into a circular hole and you know how frustrating that can be.

For example, if you're looking to integrate more exercise into your weekly routine so you can feel strong and be better equipped to take on life's everyday tasks, we have to consider many factors.

What time of day will work best based on your job, kids and other commitments?

What type of exercise do you enjoy?

How much time do you have available/are you willing to carve out for a workout?

What point in the day do you have the most energy?

Will weather impact your ability/desire to exercise?

Do you have space or equipment at home to work out?

Do you have any injuries or limitations to consider?

These are all questions that need to be answered before you just dive into the commitment of exercising more often, but I would also encourage you to think beyond the logistics.

I want you to think about:

Why is exercise important to you?

How does it make you feel mentally and physically?

What mindset obstacles might you need to overcome in order to ensure you follow through?

Have you had any negative experiences or thoughts tied to exercise in the past that might come up and impede your best intentions?

How do you feel about your body when you exercise?

This is the inner work that has to be done. I hope you can see the difference in the quality of the questions. It might seem silly to ask the second set of questions, but consider how many times in the past you have started an exercise regimen, only to have it slowly fade into the background. *You want this time to be different.*

Integrating exercise into your life in a way where you are doing it for the right reasons, not as a punishment, is not as simple as just starting. Especially if you want it to last. That's the key. This is why it's a little bit of trial and error because you need to experiment in order to make observations about how you are feeling with the change. Assessing whether it's working or not and what adjustments may need to be made over a period of time will allow you to really zero in on what works best for you. Remember this is all about you. If something doesn't work the first time, it doesn't mean you give up and throw in the towel. It certainly doesn't mean you're a failure. It just means you keep tweaking things until you find the right fit for you.

So if we go back to our exercise example, you might need to play with workouts in the morning, on your lunch break and in the evening. You might need to try out different types of workouts such as going to a gym, workout videos at home, using a personal trainer, joining a local workout group, or doing outdoor activities such as jogging, walking or biking. This trial and error method can take time and we aren't always as patient as we need to be, but remember you are taking into account the logistics as well as your mindset. You are looking at how you feel about yourself and what you're telling yourself as you integrate this new healthy habit into your lifestyle.

Consider the alternative though, which would be to simply dive in, get overwhelmed and then quit, over and over again. You are looking for custom solutions here that are made for you, and once you find something that sticks and that you feel good about, you will start to feel in control of the habit because you know it works for you. It certainly doesn't mean that you won't need to make changes here and there to accommodate life's twists and turns, but by the time that happens, this new habit has become so integral in your life that you won't be willing to give it up. Instead you will be open to making small adjustments to ensure it keeps working. You have to come at it from a different perspective this time and have to account for the role your mind plays because it dictates everything.

SMALL INCREMENTAL CHANGES

Throughout the process of trial and error, you need to think small. Now is not the time to think you can take on the world and do it all! Small and steady wins the race, remember? When I start working with a client, I don't go in and turn their world upside down by telling them to create balanced meals with a protein, carbohydrate and healthy fat, to start working out 4-5 days a week, to drink two litres of water a day, to get seven to nine hours of sleep, and so on.

Can you imagine? They would fire me on the spot or would begrudge the entire process!

We start small and take incremental steps forward that they truly believe they can make. Before we even do that, we have a discussion about what they've experienced in the past, what's worked and what hasn't, and why and how they feel about moving into the process of coaching. We talk about their mindset and what they are telling themselves because we both need to understand the inner obstacles we might encounter.

So, for example, if we are trying to move towards having healthier, more balanced meals be part of their routine, we might just start with breakfast. We discuss what their current breakfast routine is, how they feel about it and where there are opportunities to make changes they can feel good about. We brainstorm various options and take time to ensure they understand the components of creating a healthy breakfast so they fully understand why we are putting certain foods together. We don't talk about lunch, dinner or snacks because it would be far too overwhelming. We stick with this small step and allow time for them to adapt and see how they feel about the change. They will work on making the changes to their breakfast over a period of time and once they feel they have a good handle on it and are feeling confident, only then do we move on to another meal. The options for breakfast are based on their likes and dislikes, their budget, what their lifestyle allows for in the morning and what will make them feel good about their choices. It's all about the client.

I worked with a client whose evening snacking had become an obstacle, as her tendency was to completely overindulge in unhealthy choices and portion sizes on most days. It was becoming detrimental to her physical and mental health, but the challenge was how to change the behaviour without her feeling as if we were taking something away that she valued. She had attached such an importance to the evening snack even though she knew it was being used to cope with other stressors in her life. So our focus was on just doing better. Making better choices and making small, incremental changes over time so there wasn't a dramatic change that was going to have her feeling overwhelmed.

Our first step was to come up with different snack options that she could rely on that were much healthier than the chips, ice cream and chocolate she was normally drawn to. We created a big list of snack options that she actually did enjoy and would look forward to, and gave her full reign to rely on one of those options for her evening snacking. The initial goal was to avoid taking away the evening snacking altogether because we knew that she had become too reliant on that snack to go cold turkey. I told her to grant herself permission to have a snack, but to consider making a better choice with regards to the quality and quantity of that snack. We wanted to slowly remove the snack's appeal and over time, have her assess whether she actually needed the snack. To start, we would still make a snack available, but we simply replaced the snacks that had very high sugar content with snacks that made her feel better, and were still delicious, while being mentally and physically satisfying. Taking this approach allowed for her to feel in control over what she got to eat and by keeping the snack option open, she was not feeling deprived.

You want to weave healthy habits into your lifestyle as seamlessly as possible and if you're doing this on your own, look at making really small changes and progressively adding onto those changes only once you're feeling confident they will stick. It doesn't help to overwhelm yourself. Remember, you are playing for the long game. I want you to look way down the road into the future when considering making changes to your habits. Oftentimes we set goals around a vacation or special event we have planned so we end up taking drastic measures until that time arrives. But then what? You stop caring and go back to what you were doing before the vacation or event? How will that make you feel? How does that impact your day-to-day mindset regarding your health and your body?

This is why it's important to get it right by figuring out what will *actually* work for you in the long term. I understand that you want immediate results, but if you think back to what you have tried in the past, this was likely the approach you took and it hasn't worked. Eventually we want all of the pieces for good health to be there – a nutritious diet, active lifestyle, quality sleep, effective stress management and a healthy mindset. It takes time though, if you're doing it right and are continuously doing this inner work to make sure it's working for you.

Those that really know me know that I don't do anything small or half-assed. Going slow and taking baby steps are not normally in my nature. So understanding that the process of loving myself and my body required small, incremental, progressive steps was a little bit foreign to me and extremely uncomfortable. I tend to dive into things full-force with little to no thought as to whether I'm on the right path or if it's the right choice for me. Let me tell you that my husband hates this approach when it comes to home renovations because I don't like to measure, double-check or go slow. I just want to get it done!

But we aren't talking about home renovations here; we're talking about gaining a better understanding of myself and how to make changes to my habits that stemmed from a positive and healthy perspective. I have really tried to embrace this concept because I know full well that in the past, I made rash decisions to commit myself to some diet or program that had me taking dramatic steps which turned my world upside down. For a moment, I would believe I had finally found a way to lose the weight and keep it off once and for all, only to be left feeling helpless and like a failure. I was expected to change all aspects of my nutrition all at once, which was extremely overwhelming.

There was no time to adjust to the diet or slowly get used to what I was expected to do. It was all or nothing, which seemed like it was right up my alley, but boy was I wrong. Over and over again, I was wrong. I have learned that I need to build my confidence from the inside out by implementing small measures and habits, day by day, that I can live with in the long term and that will allow me to feel proud of my ability to master them. Trust me, it's the only way, if you're looking for long-term sustainability of healthy habits and appreciating your amazing body…*baby steps.*

SETTING YOURSELF UP FOR SUCCESS

The concept of trial and error and taking small, progressive steps really comes down to setting yourself up for success. You know deep down inside that starting another fad diet is simply you setting yourself up for failure because the diet isn't about *you*. It hasn't considered you, your mindset, your past or your lifestyle. By creating strategies that are all based on you and then slowly implementing those strategies, you are setting yourself up for success.

I always give my clients an example relating to sugar when we talk about setting them up for success. If I were someone who knew I needed to stop eating so much sugar because it was impacting my energy levels, my ability to make good food choices, the way my brain worked, and the way in which my body performed, and then decided to cut out sugar, that would NOT be setting myself up for success. In fact, it's quite the opposite. I know myself better than that and there is no possible way I would be willing to give up foods with high sugar content entirely. If I were to start down the path of eliminating sugar, the result would be messy. I would likely get very frustrated, I would go through withdrawal, cravings would be immensely tough to deal with, and in the end, I would likely give up and eat all the sugar I could find! Being unrealistic about how to meet your goals does nothing but waste time in getting you there. If I were to develop a more realistic plan to cut back on sugar over a period of time, I would be more likely to achieve the overall goal of cutting sugar out of my daily routine.

One of the best examples I have of setting yourself up for success is meal planning. I know what you're thinking. I hate meal planning. I don't want to spend an entire Sunday in my kitchen planning and prepping food, I have better things to do!

I'm quite sure you do and I get it.

But if we're talking about the concept of setting yourself up for success, meal planning does just that and it's a powerful tool for you to use in order to gain control over your eating habits in a healthy way. Now, while I don't want this book to be about me instructing you on how to eat or how to lose weight (that would be yet another diet and we know you don't want or need another one of those), I do have to stress the importance of meal planning and the role it can play in you feeling good about your nutrition and the way you are fueling your body.

Meal planning is a *custom* solution to ensure you are eating healthy, balanced meals that fit within your lifestyle. Nobody in their right mind wants to go through every day of their life figuring out what they're going to have for breakfast, lunch and dinner on the spot when they are hungry and busy. You know what I'm talking about.

You've had a busy day at work and get home only to realize you forgot to take the chicken out, even though you had no idea what you were going to do with that chicken. Now you are too tired to figure out what else to make, so pizza it is. Trying to come up with nutritious ideas on the spot and actually having the right foods in your home to make those meals is not setting yourself up for success. Unless you are a chef and can miraculously throw food together to create a tasty balanced meal, there has to be some planning involved. It's all about being proactive.

I often compare meal planning to heading into a meeting that you are in charge of leading. You don't just wing it and hope you will magically have amazing things to say with all your facts and information laid out for the audience. The people you are meeting with likely won't be impressed and the meeting will ultimately be a failure. The same is relevant for your meal planning. If you wake up and wing all of your meals every single day, by the end of the day you likely will not have eaten appropriate portions of protein, carbohydrates and healthy fats and will likely be left feeling unsatisfied, unorganized and unhealthy. This leads to you feeling bad about yourself and contributes to the negative internal dialogue that plagues you.

I think of meal planning as a necessary evil. If I'm being honest, I can't stand meal planning. It's a painful process trying to think about what healthy dinners my family is going to have each and every night. It can be overwhelming, time-consuming and boring.

But – it's always worth it.

By doing my meal planning and mapping out what we will have for dinner each night, I have taken the opportunity to consider what we have going on in our lives that week, which then dictates what we should eat for dinner and how much time we have to prepare and eat dinner. By being proactive, I have set myself up for success and I get to reap the benefits all week long because I know exactly what we are eating on any given day, and I know it's a reasonable meal based on what is going on in our lives that day. I have also given myself the chance to ensure I'm only buying what I actually need, that our meals will be healthy and balanced, and that my fridge and pantry have exactly the items I need to make the planned meals. I developed a game plan and now I can execute it. I'm not leaving things up to chance and hoping that within my busy day, I will have the time and mental capacity to come up with a healthy meal for my family based on the things I randomly grabbed at the grocery store. That will not happen in my household. There's a sense of control that is gained by being prepared and setting yourself up for success. There's less chance you will deviate from your plan because you've already made the decisions in advance.

So, yes, you have to do some leg work ahead of time and put some thought into what your meals will look like and what you need to make those meals come together. But when it's done, it's done. This is another opportunity for you to be selfish and make it all about you. Meal planning allows for you to make healthy meals, which ultimately will leave you feeling energized and aligned with the health goals you have set out for yourself. What you choose to eat is based on your life and what you have going on in it. It's a custom meal plan.

It's not a meal plan that some diet has given you where you dislike most of what's in it, where the meals don't fit with your schedule, where you aren't mentally or physically satisfied by the food, which you end up ditching partway through the week. No. You've taken the time and effort to map it out and set yourself up for a successful week filled with healthy, delicious meals.

NON-NEGOTIABLES

For me, meal planning is one of my non-negotiables. It's just something I'm not willing to give up no matter how much I dislike the process of coming up with dinner ideas. There's far too much benefit and value for me in the process of planning. It leaves me feeling confident knowing that I will be consuming healthy meals to fuel my body. I feel in control without feeling like I'm *being* controlled. I get to have a say and make the decisions. It can be an empowering process, especially for someone like me that relied so heavily in the past on some diet to dictate what I was allowed and not allowed to eat.

Did you notice that I haven't really mentioned the food "prep" part? Just the "planning"? I cannot and will not spend hours of time on a weekend prepping a bunch of food for the upcoming week. I prepare my overnight oats and I make a big quinoa salad or roast veggies and chicken for lunch, but that's the extent of my prepping. For me it's all about the planning piece, but if you also want to do some prep in order to set yourself up for success for the week, all the power to you!

When I say that meal planning is one of my non-negotiables, I mean it will always be part of what I do to take care of myself. No matter what. Generally, I plan on Saturdays and grocery shop and prep on Sundays, but should something get in the way of any of that, it still gets done. I just may have to shift the days around, but in the end I will always have a plan. I can't imagine trying to figure out every single day what my family would have for dinner. If they had it their way it would be tacos, pizza, burgers and takeout. Not happening on my watch. That's because those types of meals don't help me stay committed to my own health goals. They don't make me feel good physically or mentally. Yes, that might sound selfish, but if you think about it, it also benefits my family because now they too are getting healthy meals. Trust me, it's not that way 7 days a week as we generally get takeout or eat out on Saturday nights, which is a nice break for me, but the other 6 days, I have a plan that I feel good about.

To help with the process of meal planning, you can always rely on meal prep services or meal kit delivery a few times a week or month to help alleviate the load of cooking every night. Recognizing that you don't have the capacity to cook a meal from scratch each and every night is great self-care! The various services offer a variety of meals including vegetarian options, family-friendly options, and quick-cook options in which they will detail the nutritional information for each one so that you can make an educated decision. They have various packages to meet your budget requirements and you can opt in and out week-to-week to fit your schedule. I take advantage of these services one week a month when I know I have a lot on my plate. It's a huge relief and we get to try out new recipes that I can create again on my own in the future.

I dread the process of sitting down on a Saturday trying to figure out dinners, but let me tell you that when I'm done, I feel like a rock star! It's an accomplishment for me and it gives me confidence in my quest to be healthy knowing I have my meals set for the week. I'm definitely not willing to give up that feeling and that confidence, so hence the non-negotiable. I'm also a bit of a control freak so you can only imagine what meal planning does for that side of me. It's greatly satisfying and makes me feel like I've got my ducks in a row (do people still say that or is it just me?).

It's important for you to create your own non-negotiables. They're commitments you are making to yourself that are reasonable and well-thought-out. They are habits related to your self-care that you're not willing to bend on, at least not very often. Habits that you won't have a debate over in your head and that you feel so strongly about that you are willing to stick to your guns to ensure you follow through. Another one of my non-negotiables is power walking. I carve out space every single day (with very few exceptions) to power through a minimum 5km walk. I strap on my earbuds, listen to a true crime podcast and hit the pavement no matter the weather. There are no excuses and no negotiating with myself. It's just something I do because I know how great I feel physically and mentally during and after my walk.

However, just because it's non-negotiable doesn't mean I'm always hyped to do it. There are days, especially if it's raining or downright cold, where I absolutely want nothing to do with being outside, let alone power walking up and down country hills for 5km. But I do it anyway. Not because I have to or because someone told me I should, but because I value it. *I do it for me.* This is the difference from when I used to follow diets and workout programs. I was always doing things because the diet told me to, not because I wanted to or because it really worked for me.

Let's talk about sleep for a moment. Sleep is also an area of my self-care I don't compromise on very often. I value my sleep and strongly dislike feeling tired, so getting to bed each and every night between 10pm and 10:30pm is a must for me. By doing so, it allows me to get my seven to nine hours and leaves me feeling refreshed and ready to take on the day by morning. My body and mind will be functioning at their best, and being well-rested feeds the execution of the other self-care habits that are important to me.

Other people can't tell you what your non-negotiables should be. You could come up with a whole slew of habits you "should" have as non-negotiables, but remember it needs to be personalized for you in order for them to stick. These are habits you need to develop on your own and then assess the importance they have to you. Habits don't become non-negotiables overnight either. It takes time for you to understand what habits you want to stick with based on how they make you feel mentally and physically. You also need to understand what habits you are ready, willing and able to make a priority. Like I said at the beginning of this chapter, this stuff is hard, but with a little perseverance and consistency, you will stop negotiating with yourself. Of course, only after all of this inner work has been done.

SAYING NO & SETTING BOUNDARIES

Part of saying yes to yourself, whether it's with your non-negotiables or anything else, sometimes means you are saying no to other things or other people. The process of integrating healthier habits into your daily routine will sometimes require you to assess how and where you spend your time. Perhaps it's less time at restaurants or less time in front of the television. You will need to evaluate what may be contributing to poor health choices or how you are spending your time that ultimately takes you away from spending time focusing on healthy habits. It certainly doesn't mean you need to say no to things that bring you joy, but you need to find balance. As you navigate life, there will be obstacles or challenges that present themselves and it's your responsibility to decide how you proceed.

That decision will be based on the value you see in places you go, people you interact with, how you spend your time and the impact it may or may not have on your health. So if you are someone that eats out frequently, there needs to be thought that goes into the impact eating out has on your health, and more importantly, how you feel about yourself. How much do you value eating out? How do you feel after you eat out? What is the trade-off? Would anything change if you ate out less?

I don't for a second believe you need to stop living and doing the things you enjoy. The alternative is to stay at home in a controlled environment, with no external influences or obstacles, which is completely unrealistic and not mentally healthy. You can find balance and say no to what doesn't hold true value for you, and yes to what does. All while feeling like the choices you're making stem from a healthy mental position, not a position of "I can't, I'm not allowed, or I shouldn't."

This process requires you to think through situations you find yourself in and set boundaries you are ready, willing and able to live with, without feeling deprived. Once you feel deprived or frustrated by your decisions, the boundaries won't be there for long and you'll be back to the drawing board. By saying no and setting boundaries you are being honest and true to yourself about what you are willing to put up with and what you are willing to accept. You are creating expectations for yourself and creating principles to guide you, but they all stem from a place of positivity and growth. The boundaries are not put in place to box you in or take away your choices and freedoms. They are intended to create a level of confidence and belief in your own abilities. It's no longer a free-for-all, where you are left feeling lost.

If we use the eating out example again, it's important to understand that if you have a poor relationship with food, frequently eating out will likely cause you to eat things in portions that do not help you feel good. Therefore, every time you are invited out, or there's an occasion to celebrate, or you simply don't have the energy to cook at home, you need to consider how you feel about it first and the feelings that may follow. If you are setting boundaries around eating out, you would need to determine how often to eat out and where you are best to eat out. Notice that you aren't saying that eating out is no longer an option. It certainly can be. You are just putting boundaries on eating out so that you can continue to productively work towards inner peace and your relationship with food.

With everything I've mentioned in this chapter – trial and error, making small incremental changes, setting yourself up for success, creating non-negotiables, saying no and setting boundaries – it all comes back to your mindset. Every one of these areas requires thought, observation and evaluation on your part. The process of taking better care of your physical and mental health is not just about execution because execution without thought leads to observations and evaluations that will not last. When you implement a new habit, I want you to pay attention to your thoughts about that habit.

What are you saying to yourself about it?

How are you feeling mentally and emotionally about it?

How is it working for you?

How will you feel about it long term?

How confident are you feeling about maintaining it?

It's important to stay in tune with your mindset to ensure you stay on top of adjustments and tweaks that need to be made along the way. This is not about convincing yourself that something has to work. This is about considering you, your mindset and your lifestyle when integrating new habits and striving towards a goal. A change in mindset is a process that requires time, patience and kindness towards yourself. I know that will likely be the hard part, but remember the title of this chapter included the question: Are you still in? *Now you get to decide.*

Chapter 5

The Power of Choice

We have to look at choices from two different perspectives. The first is understanding that in order to feel as if we have control, or a say, we need to give ourselves choices so we don't feel boxed in. The second is recognizing that when we choose one direction, we are stepping away from another. Let's dig into both of these perspectives around choices.

Everything we do in life comes down to a choice. On any given day, you decide:

What to eat for breakfast

What to wear

What time to get up

What route to take to work

What to watch on television

What to eat for dinner

What time to go to bed

You get my point. You have choices. So when it comes to your self-care, I'm a huge proponent of giving yourself choices from which to select, so that you feel like you have autonomy over how you treat yourself and what you do to achieve your goals. This is one reason why diets don't work; they don't give you choices. You must eat in the way they dictate, exercise in the way they dictate, drink the amount of water they dictate, and so on. You don't get to choose. So you feel powerless.

Instead, I want you to give yourself choices. Healthy choices. As mentioned earlier, when I work with clients and we are discussing what to eat for breakfast, we put together a list of various options they can choose from on any given day. It's based on what they like to eat, how much time they have, where they will be eating, and what will work long term. So we brainstorm, tweak, add, and adjust until we have 5-6 solid breakfast options they're comfortable with. All options will be healthy, will include a protein, fibrous carbohydrate and a healthy fat, will be satiating, and will be appealing to the individual client. The reason for this process is to give them choices. Now they are empowered to pick a breakfast they will enjoy based on how much time they have in the morning, what they're in the mood to eat, and what ingredients they have on hand. They are less likely to stray and make a poor choice because they have already decided that the options we came up with will work for them and are appealing. They are also more confident now because they know that no matter what breakfast they choose from the list, it will be healthy and delicious and will fuel their body, leaving them feeling energized.

The same process can be said about vacations, holidays and social gatherings. We are given an abundance of choices on a menu, at the buffet, and at the dinner table. The first thing I remind clients about is that you aren't on vacation or getting together with friends and family at Christmas, for example, just to eat. That is not the purpose of vacation or Christmas. If that was the sole purpose you could have stayed home. You are going on vacation to disconnect from the day to day, spend time with those you care about, and to create experiences and memories. Not to eat. The fact that we eat when on vacation is purely out of necessity. If you took the food and alcohol away from the vacation, you would still be left with all of the other important aspects of the vacation – shopping, sunshine, culture, family and friends. Therefore, we don't need to rationalize eating and drinking in excess simply because we are on vacation. You have choices other than to over indulge. This is where the inner work comes in again. We need to consider the dialogue going on in our minds and the perspective we have about vacations and other outings.

I'm not saying you won't want to have a few piña coladas or experience the cultural delicacies while away, but we can do it in moderation while taking our health into account. We can do this with a healthy mindset. It doesn't have to be an all or nothing attitude. I encourage you to think about how you want to feel by the end of your vacation. I would imagine you don't want to feel sluggish, with an upset belly and feeling guilty about the choices you made. Then when you get home you feel as if you have to "start again." That is a diet mentality because you weren't perfect. You don't have to be perfect on vacation. It's just helpful to consider the options available to you while you're there, and consider what is of value to you from the choices you are given.

The same theory applies when we're celebrating a holiday or event. For some reason we feel this need to go all in. Overdo it. Be excessive. Eat and drink things that you really don't care for just because it's there. If you were being honest with yourself and assessed the food and drink options available to you at a gathering, chances are you don't actually LOVE them all. So pick what you actually LOVE and then enjoy it. Then move on. At restaurants you are certainly provided with an abundance of choices, so be selective. Decide where you want to indulge based on what's actually important to you. If you don't care for the bread served before dinner or having an alcoholic beverage, but you LOVE dessert, order dessert. You don't need to have the bread, alcohol AND the dessert. Be choosy. Make choices that matter to you. Keep in mind that it's only one meal, so the other meals and snacks in your day can still be aligned with your goals. You don't need to throw the towel in on the whole day or the whole weekend.

You have choices in all of these scenarios, and with some, you can even assess your choices ahead of time and make decisions before you are faced with them. Again, I want you feeling like you have a say and that you get to dictate what is going to work for you. Understanding that vacations, holidays, restaurants and other gatherings can cause your insecurities around food to present themselves, it's important to recognize that you are still in control and can gain confidence from your ability to stand strong in the choices you make.

When working with clients, we take the same approach to exercise as we do with food. We explore what it is they enjoy doing to move their body. There is absolutely no value in selecting a form of exercise that you don't enjoy. If you don't like it, you won't do it. End of story. You can try to convince yourself that because your best friend has had great success as a runner, that running will be the solution to you feeling and looking great. But you hate running. You dread running. So why would you do it? There are so many different options for moving your body that you should be able to pick a couple that will keep you active and strong because, let's face it, there are very few people that actually love working out and get excited to do it. There are a million other things I'm sure you would prefer to be doing than working out, but you need to move your body. I don't care whether your goal is to lose weight, gain weight, tone up or just be healthy, you need to be active. So pick what you love! You're more likely to stick with it.

Come up with a list of options you confidently feel you would enjoy doing, and then you pick. Maybe it's walking outside, biking, workout videos from home, hiring a personal trainer, group fitness classes, swimming, hiking, jogging, hitting the elliptical, recumbent bike or treadmill, yoga, or weight lifting. I don't care what you like or what you can see yourself doing – it's a personal decision. Remember, you get to choose because you are now doing what works for you, not what someone else told you to do. Just create your list and then pick out what activity you will engage in that day based on your energy level, how much time you have, what the weather is like, injuries you may have, and what you're in the mood for that day. The key is that you get to decide because you've given yourself choices.

As a side note, please don't believe that you need to do your exercise all at once. You can break up your exercise into smaller chunks and sprinkle them throughout your day. This can make exercise more appealing too, when you know you don't have to lift weights for an hour or go on an hour-long walk. Doing 15-20 minutes throughout your day can be very effective and much more manageable if you aren't able to carve out a long period of time all at once. Weave it in and it might feel like less of a chore. Again, you are doing what works for you and you get to decide how you're going to move your body so that you feel great, mentally and physically.

Let's step away from the concept of boxing yourself in. This is what diets do to us. Let's stop thinking you can only eat certain foods or exercise in certain ways in order to achieve success and feel great about your body. This will only bring frustration and boredom. What happens if you're boxed in for too long? You stray. You pick something else, and most times, it's not the healthy choice and doesn't contribute to your goals. There are always consequences from your choices. So by giving yourself a variety of healthy choices, whether it's for food, exercise, or methods to manage your stress, you increase the odds of the outcome being positive. You know what happens when you get frustrated by eating the same foods or doing the same workout you've done for months. You rebel. You feel entitled to have or do something different. And different often doesn't mean you pick the next best option. You go to the extreme and eat junk and protest the exercise. Neither of which have a positive outcome because now you feel crappy physically and mentally.

Now, here is where I have to admit that I don't tend to give myself a wide array of choices when it comes to my breakfast, lunch and afternoon snack. I tend to have the same thing every day, at least from Monday to Friday, but that's because it's simple and works with my lifestyle, keeps me on a path I feel comfortable with and allows me to feel confident in what I'm putting in my body. I can also do some prep in advance for the upcoming week so I don't have to make a tough choice each and every day for every single meal. I already know what I'm having for breakfast, lunch and for my afternoon snack. I've already made the decision and I stick to it. Dinner is different as I incorporate a wide variety of meals into each week and like to select choices that work for my family as a whole. I'm okay with this approach where I consistently eat the same thing throughout most of my day. I don't feel deprived or bored and this works for me.

That's what it's all about. I have found a strategy that, mentally and physically, works for me. This doesn't work for everyone which is why I encourage my clients to give themselves variety and choices if that's what will work better for them.

I take a similar approach to my workouts. I do a short strength training workout every morning before I start my day, and do a 5-7km walk taking the same route each time. I get variety in the actual exercises I perform, but I generally follow the same structure in terms of where and when I get my daily movement in. This routine works for me. It took me a long time to figure it out, but I finally landed on this strategy that has me feeling strong, healthy and confident. Again, that's what it's all about. Finding what will work for *you*. Giving yourself choices so you have the opportunity to understand yourself and gain clarity around what allows you to gain ownership over your habits.

Something else to consider when it comes to having the ability to choose what you eat is the link to your mental health. Would you make healthier choices if you knew there was a direct correlation between your food and your mental health? This connection is still being looked at by scientists but it's fair to believe that because our nutrition impacts other diseases such as high blood pressure, diabetes and heart disease, it could also impact mental health. We know that good nutrition helps with our physical health, and our physical health is connected to our mental health, so I encourage you to recognize the benefit of nutrition to your mental health. You want to feel the best you can feel in your own body, but don't you also want to feel the best you can in your own mind? I'm not saying your food choices can eliminate any challenges you experience with your mental health, but I know it to be true that when I'm eating nutritiously and making healthier food choices, I feel so much better physically *and* mentally. And remember, I work through my depression day in and day out so I feel I can speak to the impact of my food choices. It changes my outlook on the day, how I cope with stress, my productivity, and my ability to communicate and stay positive. Making healthier food choices should be aligned with your physical health goals, but considering how they're aligned to your mental health goals can take your decisions to a whole new level.

Now please know that you won't always make the healthy choice. You aren't perfect. I always encourage my clients to be present when making choices so that even if they choose the cake over the fruit, they have done so consciously, with full awareness of the impact of those choices. As a result, they are less likely to feel guilt (which is not a beneficial emotion) because they have made their choice deliberately and therefore with confidence. Then they can move on. There is no punishment the next day, extra exercise or cutting out foods. Again, that's a diet mentality. When you disconnect and simply make choices based on habit or emotion, you don't get the opportunity to understand why because you weren't paying attention. So all you are left with are questions and guilt. It's not productive. Instead, it becomes a pattern. By not stopping to think about the choices you have in front of you, you don't have to face the reasons why you continue to make the poor choices. You aren't actually facing what's going on internally and that's a dangerous place to be. Taking away the distractions like your phone and being mindful when you are presented with various self-care choices throughout the day will increase the likelihood of making the choice that leaves you feeling confident and empowered.

You also need to recognize the various emotions you experience from moment to moment throughout your day. You can drift from peace to frustration to loneliness to boredom to overjoyed to overwhelmed and everything in between, on any given day. These emotions can drive you to mindless eating in order to escape from them. You are looking for a way to disconnect from how you are feeling and food seems to provide a sense of comfort and stability in that moment. It allows you to suppress your emotions, and instead, bring temporary relief and joy by consuming foods you associate with positive feelings. In that moment, you forget and are successful in escaping reality, but the moment is fleeting. So on top of the emotions you were experiencing before you chose to eat, they are now compounded by guilt and shame. The escape was short-lived and is never worth it, yet it's another pattern and habit you continue to return to.

I understand the desire to shut your brain off and disconnect from your world even if it's only for a few minutes. It always seems like a good idea at the time and you have somehow convinced yourself that it's the solution to escaping your emotions. Having the ability to recognize this behaviour and stop it before it happens is so important, yet so difficult. We are experts in ignoring that little voice inside that's saying, "Are you sure you want to do this?" because there's another voice saying, "Yes! This will make me feel better."

If you know this behaviour is common for you, I encourage you to get comfortable confronting your emotions in the moment in order to call out why you are being driven to food. Perhaps journaling your thoughts at that moment, stepping outside into nature or engaging in a hobby will provide you with the gift of time. Time to engage in self-reflection and to recognize the emotions you are experiencing. Time to gain perspective, understand your reaction and confront the emotion in a more constructive way. And time to understand that turning to food to escape those emotions is only a temporary solution and one that will likely have additional consequences.

This whole concept of sitting with your emotions and stepping away from food takes practice and discipline, and if we circle back to giving ourselves choices, we can see their importance. By creating an environment in which you give yourself a variety of healthy food choices for moments of high emotion and ensure they are on hand and available to you, the more likely you are to turn to those choices. Even when you have an overwhelming desire to run and hide, you want to give yourself the best opportunity you can not to sabotage your health goals by making choices that aren't aligned with those goals. Give yourself a fighting chance. Take on the emotional rollercoaster and cut the tie to food. I know it's easier said than done and I know that exploring your emotions can open up a whole other can of worms and create vulnerability you aren't comfortable with. The alternative of using food as your solution to escape is also one you shouldn't be comfortable with. You owe it to yourself to provide a new set of choices as the emotional highs and lows will always be present.

The concept of *rewarding* or *treating* yourself is language that has also become prevalent within the diet industry. You are not a dog and rewarding or treating yourself based on behaviours you have exhibited is not productive. Yes, you can be proud of yourself, and yes, you can reward yourself for your efforts and success, but not with the very thing you are trying to gain control of – food. Making nutritious food choices and choosing to take better care of yourself deserves more than the reward of food.

Then there's the idea of the "cheat" day where we tend to overindulge in the food we know doesn't make us feel good. Is this helping to reinforce the behaviours and habits you are trying to alter? Or is it setting you back? I'm all for choosing a particular meal or part of a day to let go and simply consume what you feel like, whether it's a healthy choice or not. The difference here is in the approach. You aren't treating it like you've cheated or done something bad, or like you are rewarding yourself. You are simply allowing your own intuitions to guide you without any rules or deprivation. This is the opportunity to have a meal or particular food that has great value to you and that you truly enjoy, but you have consciously chosen not to make it part of your regular routine as it isn't aligned with your health goals. Do you see the difference? It's important to understand that your choice to consume a less healthy option needs to be done consciously and needs to come from a place of mindfulness and intention. Not because you feel you are deserving of it and are treating it as a "cheat", "reward" or "treat".

I have a fabulous client example to share with you that clearly demonstrates this concept of rewarding yourself via other means than food. My client wanted to set a goal for herself that was a few months into the future to give herself something to set her sights on that kept her mind in a positive place. While the ultimate goal was weight loss, we didn't set a particular number on the scale as that felt like too much pressure. Instead, she wanted to reach the goal of consistently integrating specific habits related to meal planning, exercise and making healthy food choices into her daily routine so that she remained organized and feeling her best. To many, this goal might feel vague and leave things open to interpretation, but not to my client. She knew exactly how she wanted to feel by the specific date we selected. She knew the habits she wanted to form as part of her daily routine. She knew she would be able to gauge if she had put the work in and whether she had achieved a healthy mindset around these habits. She knew herself and we created the goals based on that.

She also had a reward in place for herself. Something that had meaning to her and had absolutely nothing to do with food. New scrubs. That's right, brand new expensive scrubs. My client is a nurse and had been eyeing these scrubs for quite some time and felt that this would be a wonderful way to reward herself for the consistency of healthy habits and achieving a healthy mindset. It wasn't at all tied to weight loss and the reward was custom. It was fantastic! I was so proud of her because she was looking beyond the scale and understood the value of the reward. In case you're wondering, she got the scrubs because she crushed her goal!

It's important to understand the potential impact other people in your life can have on your choices. You can't let other people dictate how you should feel about your choices or dictate what the choices are that you should actually make. As mentioned earlier, those around you will often encourage you to skip your workout, eat the dessert, stay up late, or drink the alcohol, just so they can feel better about the choices they are making. They don't have your best interest at heart and if they did, they would say nothing in regards to you making healthy choices that serve you. In my experience, sometimes other people can't wrap their heads around why you would want to make the healthy choice when you have other choices available to you. They feel that because they would be depriving themselves by making those healthy choices, you must feel that way too. You are in charge and not accountable for alleviating their guilt and making them feel better about their choices. Your choices don't impact them. They are accountable for their own choices so I encourage you to stand in your own strength and remember why you are making the choices you are.

I would also encourage you to slow down, be present, recognize that you have choices, if you've given yourself some, and choose deliberately based on what it is you want for yourself. Consider having a journal that contains a list of the various choices you have given yourself. A list of ways you enjoy moving your body, a list of healthy go-to snack options, a list of stress reducing activities, a list of your go-to people for support. By having your choices written down, you will have direction in the moments where life gets crazy or emotions may take over. Visualize your choices and how they might play out. Choices are empowering and allow you to own the process. Choice equals freedom. You get to decide. Not some stranger that knows nothing about you like when you sign up for another diet.

Not only do you have to give yourself choices, you have to take responsibility for the choices you ultimately make. When you finally take responsibility, you are then empowered to make different choices. Better choices. Healthier choices.

So the question becomes: *Are you going to choose differently?* It's up to you. Nobody else. And that can be daunting.

I read a quote that I found to be so powerful that I wanted to include it here. Please read it several times and let it sink in.

"Getting your shit together requires a level of honesty you can't even imagine. There's nothing easy about realizing you're the one that's been holding you back this whole time." - Jayde

Wow, right?

When you choose to skip your workout, order in rather than cook, or stay up late to finish a movie when you have work the next day, do you think you're avoiding the hard work? Possibly. Or perhaps making these choices on a not-so-great day *is* self-care. You have to assess the difference and trust yourself to make decisions that are in alignment with your goals. You know it's so much easier to order in, skip your workout and stay up late watching movies. But are you letting yourself off the hook? You also know how after a crappy day, it can be tougher to make a home cooked meal, do your workout and head to bed early. But then the question becomes: Are you pushing yourself too hard? At that moment, you are empowered to choose. There will always be consequences to your choices and as long as you are honest with yourself, you will be able to make sound decisions regarding your self-care habits.

Something to consider if you find yourself backing out of your self-care commitments is how you spend each and every minute of your day. Do you think you could have cut out things that truly aren't serving you, yet you did them anyway? Likely. So the time and energy you put into tasks like those take time and energy *away* from actions and behaviours that could have served you better. You may be doing this day after day and perhaps now is a good time to begin reflecting on how you spend your time and what you put your energy towards.

Here's another quote I wanted to share with you. It's short, to the point and extremely powerful. Read it and read it again. And then again.

"Whatever you are not changing, you are choosing." – Laura Buchanan

So when you don't make changes, even when you know you need to for the greater good of your physical, emotional and mental health, you are *choosing* those habits and behaviours. It hurts to even write that because I know that I chose that for a very long time, yet continued to play the victim. I see clients make unhealthy choices every day because they aren't ready to do the hard work. The inner work. It's not good enough to say, "I want to lose weight." I said that over and over for many years, I suppose, hoping something would magically change if I said it enough. As the saying goes, actions speak louder than words. You might think you want it, but by continuing to avoid the hard work and make choices that don't align with what you say you want, you are *choosing* the opposite of what you want. So then I guess you can't complain, right? We can't continue to play the victim. Me included. We would rather ignore the pain or underlying root issues that continuously overshadow our good intentions, than make the tough choices.

For some reason, I don't have a lot of vivid memories from my childhood, but I know it was wonderful, with amazing experiences and a close-knit family. Yet if you were to ask me to recall certain memories, I have difficulty with that. So when I think back about what could have shaped my thoughts and beliefs concerning my body, my poor relationship with food and the lack of self-confidence and self-worth I have struggled with for most of my adult life, I'm sort of lost. I know that my mom always had challenges with her weight and tried various diets throughout my childhood, and my dad didn't have the healthiest of eating habits. There was always an abundance of junk food in the house and I also don't recall ever being talked to about healthy eating and a positive body image. But do all of those things equate to the unhealthy relationship I developed with food and the extremely poor body image that resulted? Has it shaped the choices I make related to my self-care? I have no idea. It's not that I'm looking for someone to blame, because I'm not. I often wonder how this happened and where it stemmed from as I would love to gain some clarity. At the end of the day, I am accountable for my choices and the way in which I take care of myself.

I do strongly believe that once we acknowledge that by not changing, we are choosing, we just might be able to move forward.

You always have a choice to show up. Now you have to own it. You know that making the healthier choice is always worth it. Nobody ever finishes a workout and thinks "I wish I hadn't done that workout." That would be ridiculous! So I encourage you to explore self-destructive behaviours and be present when you are faced with a choice that impacts your physical and mental health. Let's come off autopilot and stay tuned into the decisions you are faced with because next time, *you just might make the better choice.*

Chapter 6

Unsubscribe from
The Diet Mentality

Everywhere you look there's promotion around a diet or some sort of gimmick for losing weight; whether it's on television, social media, in magazines or on the radio. Big promises that make it sound simple, feeding into your desperation to lose the weight and feel great in just a few short weeks with just a few simple steps. They tell you what you want to hear and because you are vulnerable, you often fall for it.

How hard could it be? You ask yourself.

Maybe this is the diet that will finally work. Maybe this is what will allow me to love my body again.

They tell you the easy parts of the diet and leave out the most important parts like the impact it will have on you mentally and emotionally. They don't address that aspect. They don't care that this isn't your first rodeo and you've been down this path before. They try telling you this time will be different, and you're buying what they're selling because you don't know where else to turn to or what else to try. I can't say I blame you.

These promotions were very overwhelming for someone like me who so badly wanted to lose weight. It provoked a glimmer of hope. A feeling of "what if?". A thought that maybe this time would be different.

One of the most dramatic diets I ever got sucked into was Dr. Bernstein. Even as I talk about it, it's almost like having an out-of-body experience. It's as if I'm talking about somebody else's life, not only because it was so long ago, but because I still can't fathom that I was a willing participant. Thinking about the state of mind I must have been in to believe it was a good idea to put myself in that situation is extremely concerning, but I was desperate and this is what these diets capitalize on.

I was the mom of a young child and had gained quite a bit of weight during pregnancy that I was still struggling to lose, all while being a busy professional in the corporate world. I felt that I needed that weight gone and was feeling extremely insecure at the time. A feeling that was all too familiar. It was daunting trying to figure out how I was going to get the weight off, and knowing, of course, that my self-esteem was so closely tied to my weight. So I made the decision to commit to the Dr. Bernstein weight loss program and it ended up consuming my life.

I was required to go into their location every week to weigh in and meet with someone that worked there to get a needle in my ass

(I can't even remember what was in that needle) and then be judged based on whether or not I had lost weight that week. I remember not enjoying what I was eating or even being satisfied by the food, and there certainly wasn't a whole lot of it being consumed. But that shouldn't be surprising. I was given a list of foods I could eat, with specific brand names, and don't remember ever being told why I was to eat these foods. Never did they ask me how I was feeling mentally or emotionally, but I guess that's not very surprising either considering the staff employed there were stoic at best.

Due to the fact that my mental health was never considered, the chronic dieter in me found a way to beat the system. A way to lose weight on weigh-in day while still managing to get my food fix each and every week. It should have been the telltale sign that this was yet another diet that wasn't going to work for me. I wanted to lose weight so badly, but really wasn't willing to conform to everything because I felt deprived. It wasn't a diet that was made for me.

Throughout the week, I would weigh myself every morning at home to make sure I wasn't gaining and hoped I was managing to lose from one day to the next. By the time I was ready for my weekly weigh-in at the office, there weren't any surprises. For the most part, I was successful each and every time I went for my weigh-in and it was amazing how confident that made me feel. I was proud of myself. The way I felt about myself was directly related to what the number on that scale said.

My trick to circumvent the system was to schedule my weigh-ins at 7:30am on Fridays before I headed to work; it would give me the opportunity to have a "free" day of eating whatever I desired and craved. My next weigh-in wasn't for another week, so I would have plenty of time to get back on the diet and wouldn't have to pay a price on the scale for my day of indulging. While my end game was definitely to lose weight, a big focal point for me was going to work knowing I could consume a bunch of crap all day long. We had a cafeteria there so I would buy breakfast, lunch and two oversized cookies, which was something I didn't get to do any other day of the week. I felt free. I wasn't restricted. Everything tasted so good.

That feeling didn't last long though. By the time Friday afternoon came around, I was in the washroom and in agony. It was clear that my body was rejecting the type and amount of food I had consumed that day. I felt physically awful, but it didn't stop me from doing it week after week because mentally I loved it. I loved having anything I wanted to eat without feeling deprived and I now had full control over what I got to eat instead of this awful diet dictating my choices.

I was very successful with Dr. Bernstein in terms of meeting my goal to lose weight, but let me tell you, I was miserable. It consumed my life, my every thought and every decision. I ended up losing far too much weight, to the point where I had people questioning whether or not I was anorexic. Obviously, I wasn't willing to maintain this lifestyle because it got far too expensive and was just impossible for me to maintain this way of eating. We aren't intended to put our minds and bodies through this type of deprivation and punishment. The fact that I was a willing participant for many, many months demonstrates my level of desperation and what I was willing to do in order to be smaller in a quick period of time. I certainly didn't learn anything about proper nutrition, exercising, adequate sleep, staying hydrated or anything else related to properly taking care of myself. The only thing I learned was how to follow a meal plan that I had absolutely no say over and that deviating from that plan would result in failure. I can't even wrap my head around what sort of havoc that diet played on my body, let alone the impact it had on me mentally.

When you see ridiculous ads that say "Lose 16lb in 2 weeks!" What's your initial response? Mine is to roll my eyes (it wasn't always though), but if you're still at the point where you are curious, this tells me you are still willing to believe that quick fix diets and programs are what you deserve. It means you still think it's possible and it just might work for you. It likely means you are a serial dieter and when one diet doesn't work, you put all of your hope into another one. And the cycle repeats. The thing I want you to think about when you see an ad like this is what comes after the 2 weeks? What are you supposed to eat when they stop telling you what to eat? What is this teaching you about food? If you're able to last the entire 2 weeks, you will likely lose weight, but what will happen to your weight after you return to your regular eating habits? You know the answer. Then you start again from scratch, searching for another gimmick that has you taking drastic measures and taking on a mental load so large that it's not sustainable.

Let's stop the cycle.

You've bought into the hope that these programs will be life changing and all you've really received in return is less confidence, more frustration, and a messed up metabolic system. Let's also not forget about the money you invested in the various diets, gimmicks and programs. I can't even think about what I've spent or it'll make me sick. The confusion heightens every time you try something new because each and every program has a different philosophy. No carbs, high fat, low fat, high protein, counting macros, measuring food, counting calories and on and on. How are you supposed to keep track, let alone know what is actually correct and healthy? These programs simply *tell* you instead of *educating* you. So then when you're left to your own devices, you have no idea what you should eat, why you should eat it and in what portions. On top of that, you continue to compound the body image concerns and lack of self-worth. I don't question why you can't stick with these programs, I question why you would!

What about the other aspects of self-care that can impact your ability to lose weight and feel good about yourself? Exercise, sleep, stress management, hydration, inflammation, hormones and mindset, just to mention a few. These are not talked about or considered, which should immediately cause you to throw up red flags. There is no big picture thinking with diets or full circle approach, and they certainly don't consider you, your story or the inner work that needs to be done.

So the question becomes:

How do you unsubscribe from the diet culture and mentality?

Especially when it's been so ingrained into your mind. Especially when you've had previous success - no matter how short lived it was.

For some reason you think this time it will be different.

I hate to break it to you – *it won't.*

You have to recognize what you've been doing to yourself each and every time you start and stop a new diet. What you have done to your body and your mind. It's a cycle and it has to stop. This is an opportunity to say NO. Remember how we talked about saying NO to things that are no longer serving you? This is one of those things. You have to decide that you will *not* start another diet, no matter how appealing or promising it may seem.

Diets are restrictive and as stated earlier, are not designed for *you*. Their primary focus is to make you smaller. Nothing deeper than that. Even though you will initially have positive results when starting a diet, it won't be long before you are fed up and return to old habits. It's not sustainable. In the past, have you questioned why you start and then stop? Even when it's working? Why would you stop a diet that's doing what it's intended to do? The answer is likely because you know you can't maintain it long-term. You just can't picture yourself doing whatever unsustainable things they have you doing, forever. That's the sign you've been looking for. You know deep down inside it's not for you. That's because it's *not* for you.

Oftentimes when I'm working with a client, I have to stop a session to ask them:

How's that working for you?

When I ask, I mean it sincerely and honestly, totally without judgment, and not sarcastically. It provokes thought and conversation. It's a powerful question to ask yourself and it deserves an honest answer.

I once had a client that came to me desperate for help. She was in the midst of doing some sort of crazy group workout program and was on a diet where she had to eat chicken and broccoli for breakfast and all sorts of other ridiculous restrictions. She was miserable. She hated everything about the workouts and the diet. She had gone to these extreme measures because she was lost and felt hopeless. She got sucked into thinking these programs would be the answer, only to find out they would have the opposite effect.

I asked her: How's that working for you?

Obviously the answer was that it wasn't. Not even close.

Now this was a pretty extreme example, but asking this question can be very helpful in determining if you are on the right path with your self-care. Even when I'm working with a client and we're trying out some new strategies, I ask this question to ensure they are comfortable and confident. If they don't believe it's working or will work long-term, we shift gears. We try something different. We work on it until it clicks and they feel empowered by the change. Unfortunately not all of my clients are patient enough to stick it out until we figure out all of the pieces and that's usually because they are stuck in the diet mentality of wanting a quick fix. I can't always change that for them and they have to come to that realization on their own. In the meantime, they will continue to try new gimmicks, ignore their situation, or simply degrade themselves, but not make any progress forward. They aren't quite ready to do the inner work.

One of the first things I ask my clients when they start working with me, especially when their goal is weight loss, is what will *actually* change if they were to be successful in losing the weight. The reason I ask is because I want them to realize that we can lose the physical weight, but if we don't expose the inner root issues that cause us to hold on to the weight in the first place, the cycle will continue. Clients will often relay to me that they believe there will be an increase in their energy levels, self-confidence and productivity if they were to lose weight. I then encourage them to imagine what could happen if, instead of weight loss being the primary goal, having more energy, confidence and productivity were their primary goals. Imagine the shift in the mindset.

It's interesting because during all of the years where my weight continued to go up and down, trying different diets and not being satisfied with how I looked or felt, it always felt good when someone would compliment me on how I looked. This is what the diets ingrained in me: What did my outside look like and what changes were taking place while on the diet? At the end of the day, how others viewed my external being still didn't fix how I felt about myself. It couldn't take away my ability to find the flaws, I still had deep internal wounds, and I still couldn't be happy with how I felt about my body, no matter what size I was at the time.

Looking back, even when I actually did look great and met my personal definition of strong, healthy and fit, there was something still missing. There was still a disconnect between what was going on in my mind and what was actually true about my own body.

It has since become glaringly obvious that it doesn't matter what size or shape you are, what size clothing you can fit into or what other people think, it's truly all about what you think and how you feel internally about yourself for real change to take place. This can be a tough concept for me to wrap my head around on a consistent basis because in the past, I placed so much value on the number on the scale, how I looked and what others thought, that I tended to dismiss or forget the inner work that constantly had to be addressed. I needed to remember that the inner work impacts the outer results. For a long time I didn't even consider how my thoughts and feelings about my body were impacting the choices I was making. I was simply looking for a quick fix. For something or someone to change my outside without having to do the work on the inside, when in fact, this is completely backwards. I now know that changes to the outside will naturally come as I make changes to the inside.

My desire is to have you be honest with yourself about diets. You have to understand that, no matter how good it seems, it's not worth it and it won't work long-term. Not without considering the impact of your mindset and not without doing a deep dive into what your thoughts and feelings are around all aspects of your self-care. I'm sure there will be many out there who would love to debate this as they've had success and would claim they are happy on their diet. My hope for them is that it lasts.

Once you can let go of the hope you place on the diet industry and the hope that there has just got to be something out there that will work for you, the less power it will have over you. Once you decide to see those commercials and social media ads for what they really are, you will then empower yourself to go about being healthy in a different way and your perspective will change. Tailoring your social media feed to include individuals and organizations that are empowering, diverse and positive can be a wonderful first step. You may also want to engage with a professional that will teach you what it means to eat balanced, nutritious meals that will energize your body. A professional that looks at you and your lifestyle to design custom strategies that will bring confidence and success based on a fundamental understanding of all aspects of self-care. A professional that looks at the big picture, provides flexibility and addresses the mindset piece which is so valuable to the process of loving yourself again. You need to do your homework though, in order to find this professional. I want you to start trusting yourself and demanding the best for yourself. And that starts with saying no to diets.

Chapter 7

You Are Not Alone

Did you know that, according to the World Health Organization (2016), there are about 2 billion overweight adults, and of those, 650 million are considered to be obese? The worldwide obesity rate has nearly tripled since 1975, so we are definitely not moving in the right direction. As mentioned before, this book isn't about weight loss, but it certainly is about how you feel about yourself and how you treat yourself. So regardless of whether you are part of the statistics or not, I want you to know that you are not alone in wanting more for your health.

The process of losing weight or just trying to take better care of your health can be a lonely journey. It can feel as if it's easy for everyone else to achieve success or that everyone else somehow has it all under control. We could probably say that about a lot of things whether we're talking about people's joy around their relationships, career or family. Unfortunately, we are a society that doesn't like to talk about things we are struggling with, so it creates a facade and leaves us wondering how others are so successful. I think we need to question this or at least gain an understanding that things aren't as perfect as they may seem. Social media is the perfect forum for us to create an image of how wonderful things are when they are really just snippets in time.

When it comes to how we all feel about our bodies, weight and health, there are a lot of people struggling. Struggling in silence. In my experience, it's because of the guilt and embarrassment associated with how we look or think we look, and the reasons we don't feel good about ourselves. And I'm not talking about weight here. That's not the issue. This is simply regarding how we feel about the body we live in - overweight or not. We know the ball is in our court when it comes to the actions and behaviours that are required for change to take place, but we have a hard time wrapping our heads around what to do and how to get there. Asking for help or sharing our feelings can be a tough topic to broach because we know the onus is on us.

I've always felt as though nobody ever really cared if I struggled with my weight. At least that's my perception, and therefore, my reality. So it always felt like so much to carry on my own, and to be honest, even if someone else were to have found out the degree to which I was struggling, I wouldn't have believed that they truly cared or understood. How could they? While they may have been empathetic and would have said all the right things in the moment, I would have questioned their sincerity because they are not me. They would continue living their lives and taking care of their own needs, and rightfully so. Meanwhile, I would continue to struggle. It was a very lonely place for me and is still quite painful knowing how I struggled. I know I had people that cared about me, but it was very difficult for me to grasp why. I've always disliked feeling like a burden to anyone and I think this goes back to me not believing that anyone would actually care that much for me. So why would I rely on them for help if I didn't believe they truly cared? Strange, I know, and I'm not sure where that comes from. I have to admit though, I wish I had someone constantly checking in, asking questions and staying on top of the issues with me.

My hope is that this book can serve as some sort of support system for you. I know I'm not physically there with you, but I promise I'm there in spirit. *I feel you.*

I feel like I used to struggle in silence every time I had to get prepared to visit with family or friends for some sort of gathering or celebration. How I looked to others and how I would be perceived weighed heavily on me. A lot of thought and effort went into what I was going to wear so I could look my best. Let me clarify though. I don't just mean trying to look nice like any other person would by putting on a decent outfit, fixing up my hair and makeup, and stepping outside of my "couch look". My thoughts were all related to how I could present myself so that I looked slim, aka not fat, and how I could hide the various areas of my body I had deemed to be a problem. I would change outfits several times, ask my husband how

I looked, and get myself worked up to the point of complete frustration because I wasn't able to pull off a look that met my expectations.

I know full well that the family and friends I surrounded myself with didn't care about how big or small I was and were certainly not judging whether I looked slim or overweight. I didn't do that to other people so why would they be doing it to me? Once again, these thoughts and feelings would dominate and the insecurity was almost unbearable. I certainly don't have an extensive wardrobe from which to select, but my primary thoughts when I put on an outfit, whether it was something casual, dressy, a bathing suit, or anything in between, were always: Does this make me look fat? Is this outfit hiding my stomach? Do my arms look big? It was an exhaustive process, mentally.

I found myself more focused on my body image than my relationships, and making memories with the people around me. As you can imagine, it was not a fun way to live. Although I did appreciate these things, I was still "obsessed" with how I looked. So it makes me wonder how much of my "self-care" was for other people rather than myself. I always want my clients, those I care about, and everyone reading this book to be taking care of themselves *for themselves*. At the end of the day, you are the one that has to live in your body, and your opinion and perspective about yourself is truly the only one that matters. I can say that out loud, I can say that to other people and I firmly believe it, yet sometimes that doesn't translate to how I feel about myself. Yes, I want to do this for myself, but I have to admit there's a small part of me that still does it for other people so they have a positive opinion of me. It can be, at times, very heavy to deal with and very disempowering. I guess you would call this needing validation or approval from others, and again, I'm not sure where that comes from but it's frustrating as hell.

It's heartbreaking not only for me, but for others who feel the same way. I understand that we all like to look our best and feel good as we head out the door. I want that for you. I want you to stand proud in your body and own it and not care what others think of you. I also know that when you've lived your whole life considering the thoughts of others, it can be tough to get past. But not impossible.

Believe me when I say you are not the only one struggling. You are not the only one trying to figure out how to eat better, how to get motivated to be active, how to get better quality sleep and how to manage all the stress. You're not the only one that wants things to be different, that wants to be able to accept your body and love yourself, but doesn't know how to get there. You are not alone. This isn't about misery loving company. It's about understanding that this topic of how to take better care of yourself with a healthy mindset is a worldwide issue that impacts millions, yet we all continue to struggle internally and beat ourselves up for not being able to figure it out on our own.

This is where sharing your experiences, thoughts and feelings are important. Allowing yourself to be vulnerable and admitting that you need help can be a great starting point in moving the needle. I want to encourage you to stop struggling privately. This can be a dangerous thing when you live inside your own head, spinning, wondering, questioning, doubting, hoping, and ultimately going nowhere. Not making any progress at all. There's no one handing out shiny gold stars for doing this on your own. By opening up to a friend, family member, co-worker, coach, therapist or whoever else you trust, you are letting go of the heavy burden you continue to place on yourself. Now you can be open, honest and begin to move forward. Suddenly there's conversation. There's sharing of experiences, ideas, accountability, feedback, support, guidance, new perspectives, and potentially, change.

A few years ago, I reached a point where my weight had been creeping up gradually and I was feeling unhealthy and tired. My back hurt, my clothes didn't fit, and my confidence was shot. I knew things needed to change and even though I did this for a living, I was stuck in a place where the process of making those necessary changes was very overwhelming. I was living inside my own head and telling myself things that just weren't true, and as a result, I doubted my ability to make consistent changes. Over time, I started to confide in two close friends from different parts of my life, and through that discussion came confidence. I wasn't alone in this anymore. They were struggling too, and wanted to make some changes as well. Although we each had different approaches that we believed would work for us, we could still share our thoughts and experiences. We could share recipes, snack ideas, workout videos and strategies, and could be a voice of reason for each other. There was a sense of accountability with these partnerships, without there being pressure. We weren't making changes for each other or to please each other, we were doing it in conjunction with one another.

Having that sense of support and camaraderie was always running in the background of the work I was doing. Things started to change with my nutrition and how I was fueling my body, the workouts I was engaging in, the way I was speaking to myself and most importantly, I finally started to believe I could do what was needed to take good care of myself and feel amazing. Now, you could argue that I would have come around to all of this on my own without the support of my friends, but I'll tell you it wouldn't have been the same. I've done it many, many times on my own, in secret, trying a new diet or program and it's lonely. It never lasted.

This time was different for a variety of reasons, but having the support of two confidants was vital to my success. I wasn't alone and I had the opportunity to share my success as well as my frustrations. They kept things in perspective for me, not allowing me to go too far down the negative path when things weren't going just as I thought they should. I knew what needed to be done and still struggled. I'm human. My friends knew that and supported me regardless of the fact that I coach on these very issues for a living.

Let me reiterate that I do this for a living.

It's still hard. I had the information, the knowledge, and the expertise.

And I played the games. You know the games I'm referring to. The games related to food. I'll give you an example of a game I used to play frequently back in the day. When my family members were not around, I would see it as a prime opportunity to indulge in food I had been craving. I would almost get excited knowing they would be gone and it would give me free rein to eat uninterrupted. I would open the cupboards and the fridge to see what I could find and would start eating before I even sat back down. It could be chips, my kids' chocolate covered granola bars, fishy crackers, leftover Halloween candy, or anything else that would catch my attention. I would continue to do this over and over again hoping that each time I returned to the kitchen, I would find something to satisfy me. Not to satisfy me from a hunger perspective, because I was rarely actually hungry. There was something else that needed to be satisfied and, at the moment, food seemed to be the answer.

I wouldn't just eat one thing and be done. I would grab one small thing, sit down, inhale it and then on the next commercial break or when I couldn't resist it anymore, I would return for something else. This would carry on for 30 minutes or more. Because no one was there to witness it, it was as if it wasn't happening. I wouldn't have anyone there to question me or judge me. Mindful eating was not on my radar, and to be honest, I would scarf the food down before I was able to even recognize what was happening, which is why I continuously went back for more. I wasn't present. I wasn't aware of the chewing, the taste, the texture or the smell and certainly wasn't paying attention enough to enjoy what I was eating. I was just going through the motions of eating. Eating without paying attention resulted in me almost forgetting that it had taken place, so back to the kitchen I would go. The satisfaction I gained from the food was short lived and was soon replaced by feelings of extreme guilt and shame, and me questioning my choices. This was the epitome of self-sabotaging behaviour and I would engage in these tendencies time and time again.

As I reflect back, it's so interesting to note that I was able to justify this behaviour and had somehow convinced myself that the food would make me feel better. Had someone been home, though, I never would have followed through. I'm not sure where this justification to eat when others weren't around came from, but for some reason it felt good, and it was exciting in the moment. It was almost as if I was getting a high from it. I'm embarrassed to think that I did this, but even more than that, it confused me. It's as if one side of my brain knew what I was doing was unhealthy and understood that my actions weren't aligned with the goals I had for myself. The other side of my brain, the overpowering side it seems, didn't care and wanted what it wanted.

Due to the fact that I was constantly depriving myself, I certainly wasn't content with the choice I made to eliminate certain foods from my diet. The lifestyle I had stipulated for myself was constantly coming back to haunt me, not to mention the fact that had I been nourishing my body with what it needed, I likely wouldn't have had the need to mindlessly overindulge. The unhealthy mindset that was created by diets via food rules and regulations provoked the playing of games.

Another troubling piece to this behaviour was that I believed I would be letting other people down or be negatively judged by my actions if they were to see me indulging. That's not something that sits well with me. It's the people-pleasing perfectionist in me. So I suppose that by hiding my behaviour, I wouldn't have to face the disappointment head on. Trust me, though, there was enough self-disappointment to go around. It's difficult to grasp why the simple act of eating would foster shame and embarrassment, but it definitely speaks to this expectation I had of myself to be perfect.

I frequently hear stories of people playing the game where they justify eating junk food because they worked out that day, even though they know damn well they can't outwork a poor diet. Even just the fact that food is a constant thought in our minds and that it tends to dominate our world is a concern. I found myself constantly thinking about when I got to eat next, what I would eat, when I got to eat out next, and how I could get away with eating all that crap. All very unhealthy thoughts. At the end of the day, any games you play with yourself around food that justifies you eating poorly and more than you need represents an unhealthy relationship with food.

It's a coping mechanism or a way to deal with other issues that are actually at play.

I believe that being mindful is the first step to addressing this issue. Paying attention to what it is you're telling yourself is vital. Documenting it, verbalizing it and sharing it will make it real. It will shine a light on something you have tried to hide or bury and will give it less power. This can be done via journaling, voice notes or confiding in a friend, family member or professional therapist. Engaging in activities that you gain joy and worthiness from such as joining a sports team or a community involvement project, can also provide you with an opportunity to spend down time in a more constructive way.

Remember, I'm not a psychologist or anything of the sort, but I have played these games, justified my thoughts and behaviours, and have also seen my clients do it time and time again. It's not something that has recently developed in us. It usually stems from years and years of unhealthy thoughts and actions around food, and as a result, it creates this story that we drag along with us everywhere we go. This isn't something that is cured overnight. It takes time, patience and dedication to change. The acknowledgement of the behaviour is the beginning of your journey. Everyone has to start somewhere. The deeper learning and healing will come over time and will likely require additional outside help.

I'm at a point where I don't need to rely on my support system as much as I once did for this journey but I know they are there, and there's reassurance in that. Finding and building your support system, whether it's with one other person or a community of people, can be empowering, because not only are you getting something from it, you might just be able to help someone else in the process. There's something to be said about being a part of something. It's that feeling of inclusion and being part of a team, even if the team is only made up of two people.

When I work with my clients, we create a partnership. We are in it together. There's a relationship that's built based on trust, respect and understanding. We share with each other; not just them with me, but me with them. I share my experiences and my ups and downs with my own weight, body image and relationship with food. It's real and raw. Although we live very different lives and can be very different people, the emotions and internal dialogue is often very much the same. This allows for the right questions to be asked to ensure we are addressing the real issues and creating strategies that will work long-term. The discussion is about real life, what is being thrown at us and expected of us, and how we are dealing with it. It's quite the experience.

Finding the right person or people to provide you with this relationship is vital. You don't need to do it on your own and will likely be more successful if you don't do it on your own. Like I say to my clients, you don't need to be on an island all by yourself working through the issues on your own when I'm right here. It gives them permission to reach out, to rely on me and to avoid feeling alone. It's strange how we feel the need to do these things on our own. Maybe we feel weak if we have to rely on others or that people will question why we aren't capable of doing it on our own. I'm not sure. I do it all the time. I have plenty of people around me consistently offering to help with various things, and nine times out of ten, I don't take them up on their offer to help. People want to help. I love to help others as it gives me a sense of purpose and feels like I'm making a difference. A client once told me to give other people the opportunity to help you; you both benefit from it. It's so true. Yet when it comes to issues around weight loss, body image, or our mental and physical health, we tend to keep it bottled up and buried.

In my personal experience, keeping it all to yourself can greatly impact your mental health. The pressure you put on yourself to be successful at all "the things" is unrealistic and unhealthy. You have to be kinder to yourself and more understanding. That doesn't mean you don't hold yourself to account and don't keep the expectations of yourself high, it just means you are being realistic about what's attainable. What you say to yourself and how you say it, becomes your perception and then your reality. So that self-dialogue needs to be analyzed to ensure it's moving you in a constructive direction that is aligned with your goals. This is where another person can help you. They can offer another perspective or can point out where you aren't being fair with yourself. Oftentimes they see things you don't because you're too close to your thoughts and the situations you find yourself in. It could be the smallest idea or suggestion that could shed light on something big you have been struggling with that could make an impact.

We have to be open to new ideas and different perspectives, and step away from the narrow- minded thoughts we often have around how to improve our health. It's not always black and white, but sometimes we've convinced ourselves that the process of making change is far too daunting and we end up making a "mountain out of a molehill". Others can often kick down that mountain to expose the molehill, and suddenly, it's not so scary.

You owe this to yourself.

To open up, be vulnerable, share, and get out of your own way. It's ok to ask for help when you're struggling with your weight, body image, self-worth or any other area of your self-care.

Give this to yourself.

You likely give so much to your family, friends, children, career, and community, but cut off the giving part when it comes to you and your health. We have to stop ignoring it and start embracing it. Reach out to someone and start the conversation. Get the ball rolling and remember you are not in this alone and you are not the only one struggling.

Chapter 8

Moving Forward

We often hear and talk about this concept of motivation and assume it's something that is either naturally occurring or something we have to try to muster up. I often get asked how I stay motivated to work out or eat healthy on a regular basis, and my belief is that we put far too much stock in motivation. It's as if we think it should be a feeling that just magically appears within us, and as a result, we will automatically be driven to take better care of ourselves. The problem with this concept is that there will always be challenges and obstacles in your life that impede your so-called motivation. Then what? Do you lose your motivation and your reason for taking care of your health? Do you just hope that the motivation will eventually reappear and you'll jump back on the bandwagon? If you're clear about your purpose and your why, then your motivation will rarely waver.

It can't be about motivation, and you absolutely can't rely on it. This is where discipline enters.

We as a society are not disciplined enough to stick with habits even when times get tough. We give up and wait for motivation to kick back in. The problem with that approach is that you could be waiting for a very long time. You need to explore the level of discipline you are applying to your self-care habits and assess where you are falling short. This is where that inner work comes into play, once again. We've discussed holding yourself to a higher standard, and in order to maintain that level, you need to have discipline. It feels like such a tough word with a negative undertone, but when you truly think about the meaning and concept of discipline, it makes sense why it's so important.

If you have goals you are working towards, it really doesn't matter if you're motivated. What matters is if you are disciplined enough to follow through on the commitments you have made to yourself. You still have to do the work. Once you start to implement discipline towards your habits on a consistent basis and start to reap the rewards, this is where motivation enters the picture. You start to get excited, start to feel better, start to recognize the value of the discipline because it's starting to pay off. You then start to create momentum which allows you to continue to push forward regardless of what life throws at you. It doesn't mean it's going to be perfect, it just means you'll be consistent and won't be so willing to throw in the towel when life gets tough. You will be disciplined enough to keep going, the motivation will grow and momentum takes over. Seems like an easy process, right? Nope.

The discipline piece requires time and patience. Both of which we often lack. We want instant results, and for some reason, believe that just because we've been "good" for a short period of time, we deserve the results. We forget all about the fact that we haven't been "good" for a consistent enough period of time. We have short term memories. So when we don't see the reward from our effort, we get frustrated and quit, when, what we really need is to stay disciplined in order to keep moving forward and get over that hump. We need it long enough for the motivation and momentum to take over. Then these habits you've become so disciplined with just become part of what you do. *They become part of who you are.*

Here's another powerful quote I wanted to share with you, this time regarding discipline:

"Nobody wants to tell you why discipline is so important. Discipline is the strongest form of self-love. It is ignoring current pleasures for bigger rewards to come. It's loving yourself enough to give yourself everything you've ever wanted." – Unknown

It actually gives me chills when I read this quote, and if you are struggling with staying motivated, read it again. So when people ask me about my motivation, I tell them I don't rely on it. I rely on discipline. That way when I have a setback, I know I still have the confidence to get up and keep trying because the discipline is ingrained in me. I discuss this topic with clients regularly. There will always be moments where they don't want to cook a healthy meal, don't want to work out, or don't want to do their meal planning.

When we focus on discipline versus motivation, we are working towards a lifestyle where, despite the fact that they don't want to do something, *they do it anyway.*

Being disciplined means you are being intentional versus strict. Making intentional choices and decisions that are aligned with your goals keeps the power and control on your side. Strict implies you are deprived and "can't", "shouldn't", or "aren't allowed" and you want a more positive perspective. If you can focus on being intentional, which is on purpose or deliberate, then you have the power to do what works for you.

If I have dessert at a family gathering, I'm doing it with intention. I have made a conscious choice to indulge in something I love, I will enjoy it and move on. There is intention behind my decision. The same goes for when I choose to say no thank you to dessert when it's offered. I'm saying no with intention because at that time it doesn't work for me or I don't value it enough to have any, versus being strict and saying no because "it's bad", "I can't" or "I'm not allowed".

I don't let myself off the hook. Very rarely, at least. But when I do, it's with intention.

You need to take the decision-making power back.

When you follow fad diets, you don't have the decision-making power because you have to be strict and abide by the rules. You don't have the autonomy to decide for yourself based on your intentions. You think you need to be strict and a rule follower, but that just boxes you in and makes you feel trapped. When you can slow down and start being intentional about your choices, you just might be surprised at your ability to trust your body to know what it needs.

I know the reaction that some of you will have is to believe that it's easy for me. You will think this is what she does for a living, that you're not like that and it's so much harder for you than it is for me. That's not at all true. I haven't always been like this. In fact, it's only been over the past few years that the light bulb has gone on and I've gotten to know myself, what works for me, how to keep my head on straight, and keep fighting for what I want. Trust me I still have my tough days. It would be so much easier to just eat the crap, sit on the couch, not plan anything and simply wing it all. That would be dangerous though and a very slippery slope.

This is why you need to aim for consistency, not perfection. I have spent most of my life trying to ensure that everything is perfect and that's a very difficult expectation to meet. So when I work with clients, we aim for consistency which allows for mistakes, obstacles, downtime and grace with ourselves. It simply means that more times than not, you are implementing your healthy habits. You take the pressure off of feeling you need to be bang on with every single habit, every single day. That's what diets are all about. You need to be pretty near perfect or you fail. That's not what we're talking about here. If you can constantly remind yourself that being consistent means you are simply aiming for better in all you do, you will make progress. When I say, aiming for better, it means incrementally better, at a pace that works for you. I always give the silly example that if you eat 5 cookies every day and one day you decide to only eat 4 cookies, that's better. You get what I mean. If you were to continuously make *better* choices in the areas of nutrition, exercise, sleep, stress-management, hydration and mindset work, imagine what could happen. Over time, great things could happen.

When I'm working with a client, my goal is not to come in and turn their world upside down by barking out all the things they need to change immediately. They would be completely overwhelmed. So instead, we make small changes and continue to aim for better, week after week. We aren't looking to correct everything all at once or take on big dramatic changes. We're looking at creating the habits first, and from there, we gradually zero in on cleaning those habits up. During this time, we need to consider what's going on in their lives, where they're at mentally and emotionally, and assess what they are capable of doing right now. I encourage them to be honest and meet themselves where they're at. Sometimes we need to back down a little and sometimes we are good to push forward. It can be a balancing act, but the ultimate approach is to maintain consistency, even if that means we don't add anything to the to-do list for the time being. Knowing when to add and when to pause is important. We don't take steps backwards, but we might change our approach or just hit the pause button to honour where they're at and what they are ready, willing and able to do at that particular time. Consistency doesn't mean you give 100% every day. Consistency is being ok with a simple workout or making a simple meal on days your energy is low or you are short on time. You are still honouring the commitment you made to yourself and still building momentum.

Part of knowing when and how to move forward is trusting yourself. I will often ask my clients if they trust themselves after we've been working on a specific habit for a period of time. The answers I get are mixed, but it gives us an understanding of where we're at and how much work still needs to be done on that habit. Most times, the reason you turn to fad diets with all sorts of rules and regulations is because you don't trust yourself. You think that if the rules are outlined for you, all you need to do is follow them. Then you won't have to rely on your judgment to do what's best for you. When my clients understand that, they start to see they have a say and need to start looking internally. I want to get them to the point where they trust themselves and what they're capable of, so if we're no longer working together, they feel confident and empowered to continue their journey independently. It's an amazing feeling to watch clients learn to trust themselves.

A perfect example is when the Christmas season approaches and we talk about the steps we want to take to maintain a level of consistency. When clients say they aren't worried about it and have no intention of stopping what they've worked so hard for just because it's Christmas, I know they have reached that level of trust with themselves. It's amazing to see. They don't even hesitate. They just know it's not worth it.

They also know that it's not a straight line to success. There will be bumps and detours on the journey, but this is where discipline and consistency is key. You have to understand and appreciate that success can and will take all sorts of forms, so when you do experience it, you need to acknowledge it and celebrate it. I'm constantly pointing out even the smallest successes my clients experience because sometimes they are fixated on only the big ones. If we piece all of the small successes together, we get to the big ones and those small ones create the momentum we talked about earlier. They are the building blocks. The process is to recognize and remember the success and build on it one block at a time. I'm not sure why we seem to get hung up on the big changes because we are doing ourselves a *great* disservice when we dismiss the small wins.

If you have children, you know how important the small milestones are and how much you celebrate them. I remember when my oldest daughter took her first couple of steps and thought it was the most fabulous thing ever! I didn't wait for her to be able to run around the entire house before I acknowledged and celebrated, because I knew it was the beginning of great things to come. I wish we were better at recognizing these small accomplishments in ourselves as adults. It would allow us to trust ourselves and the process, and enable us to exhibit the patience required for real change to take place. Instead, we're more likely to be impatient, throw in the towel and come up with a laundry list of excuses as to why something doesn't work.

It's always amazing to me how quickly we buy into our own excuses as to why we won't work out that day, why we deserve that alcoholic beverage, or why we just don't have time to throw a healthy meal together. I was the queen of excuses and loved to blame everything else I could think of. I think it's time you called yourself out on the BS and started to get real. Real about what your goals are, real about what you are ready, willing and able to do in order to reach them, and real about how you are going to hold yourself accountable. This takes some soul searching, but you need to be honest with yourself. It's important to remember that your goals and self-care habits may shift and change as your health and life does. Over time, you will grow and learn from your experiences and your newfound knowledge can be applied when these changes take place.

I've worked with many clients that come to me saying they're ready to do what it takes and that they are sick and tired of feeling like they want to change. When we dive into the weeds and try to make real change, their claims fade away. It's like they've suddenly forgotten why they started this journey in the first place. Even if I'm reminding them of what they wanted out of the process at the beginning, they refuse to get real about what's holding them back. There is no accountability to themselves. There is no recognition that they are continuing to live by the excuses that hold them back, and instead of wanting to really explore how to move forward, they quit.

It's heartbreaking. Especially since I've done the same thing to myself countless times in the past. I knew what I wanted, but really wasn't willing to do what it took to get there and that's because I had never taken the time to do the inner work.

I'll tell you, I can't do it for them no matter how badly I want it for them. They have to do the work. The inner work.

On the other hand, I've had countless clients that have had the initial goal of losing weight and their primary reason for reaching out for my assistance was to lose the weight they had been struggling to get rid of for many years. They're often surprised when the weekly goals we work towards aren't specifically tied to a number on the scale. Instead, we focus on their mindset and the inner work that needs to be done in order for their behaviours and actions to change. We can only start to change their actions and behaviours when they come at it with a healthy mindset. It's so fascinating to see that, over time, without me prompting them, they start to comment more on how they *feel* than on how they look, the amount of energy they now have, the mental clarity they have or just how much their confidence has increased as a result of taking a healthy mental approach to their self-care. More times than not they end up losing weight anyway and, of course, they're proud of that, but are so much prouder of the changes they made to their mindset and the way they feel about themselves. They just love how they are now empowered and in control of the choices they are making. They recognize that it's not about a number on the scale or the size of clothing they can fit into but instead, it's about how they feel mentally and emotionally and it is amazing to witness that transformation.

For those that don't get to this transformational point, I have to admit there's a part of me that believes they blame me for it not working. I do my very best not to own those feelings though. I have worked with so many clients where it has been a success and they get to own that. They get to own the dedication, commitment and the successes they have experienced. They did it; not me.

I want you to quit the excuses and really listen to yourself. Listen to what you are telling yourself that holds you back and carve out a path forward, where you are empowered to take control of your health and the way you feel about yourself. If that means you start journaling, seek out therapy, hire a coach, join a women's group, then so be it. You just need to start before more time slips away. I want you to think about how you want to feel five, ten, twenty years from now. Not just physically, but mentally and emotionally too. Think about how you want to *feel* in your body, what you want to be able to *do*, what you want to be able to say to yourself *about* your body, and the life you want to live *inside* your body.

For me, I want to be able to travel, hike and explore the world. I want to have the energy to keep up with my grandkids and spend time in my gardens. Most of all, though, I want to have a positive and healthy mindset about the habits I've chosen to have as part of my life, and truly love myself.

Let's not take it for granted that your body will be able to keep up with the demands you keep placing on it. The everyday tasks like going up and down stairs and carrying groceries in from the car will become increasingly difficult, but you can slow down that aging process. You can take control over what the future holds by paying more attention to the present. I want you to feel fantastic in your own body today and years from now. I want you to be confident, proud and feeling your best. *What do you want for yourself?*

Chapter 9

Start Today

You don't even know how good you're supposed to feel. Our bodies and minds become used to feeling a certain way so you are no longer able to determine if you actually feel the best you can or if this is just the best you can feel based on how you treat yourself. When you start taking better care of all aspects of your health, you get to experience clarity and energy you didn't know was possible. Right now you don't know any different. You don't know that there's room for great improvement.

Where I'm reminded of this difference is when I start to slide with my own self-care. Things go downhill very quickly when, for example, I'm not eating as clean as I normally do. I experience headaches, bloating, brain fog, back aches, and depleted energy. I pay the price big time if my habits go on like this for more than a couple of days. It's as if my body is rejecting the food I've been consuming because it has absolutely no idea what to do with it. My body is sending me a message and I've learned to listen. That's not to say that I don't repeat this behaviour at various times throughout the year because, regrettably, I do. You would think I would have learned my lesson by now. Not only is my body not functioning at its best, but my mind isn't either.

I will take you back to Christmas of 2020. Due to the COVID-19 worldwide pandemic we were experiencing at the time, we weren't able to celebrate and gather with our loved ones so it was just myself, hubby and our daughters. Rather than cooking a big fancy meal, we decided to have appetizers over the course of the day. Unfortunately, this decision would end with me hunched over the toilet for most of the evening. The day started with my mom's famous banana muffins that were just loaded with sugar but were oh-so-good, and it continued with various appetizers throughout the afternoon. By the time we got to the evening, we decided to watch a Christmas movie and eat a few more munchies. It was game over for me by then. My body was sending me a message loud and clear and it was angry. My belly was unbelievably upset; I was dizzy, felt weak and thought I was going to be sick. Hubby had to escort me to the washroom where I proceeded to dry heave over the toilet and was then forced to lay down on the cold floor for fear of passing out. It was awful and it was Christmas.

My kids were down the hall wondering what the heck was wrong with their mom. No, kids. Mom doesn't have the flu. Mom just ate too much crap. This is what happens to me when I eat crappy food even for one day. Even though it was only one day, *it was all day* and there wasn't an ounce of healthy food consumed. No balance for me – I was all in. I didn't listen to my body and I should have known better. I know my body well enough by now to know it can't handle this amount of crappy food with no nutritional value. But I did it anyway. In reflecting, it was apparent that some of my old habits had crept back in and I got so caught up in the excitement of being able to eat whatever I wanted, whenever I wanted, that I failed to respect my boundaries and what I know about my body. Well – lesson learned.

It's important that we listen to our body and the cues it sends. It won't lead you astray when it comes to your hunger and fullness. Being in tune with your body can be difficult but very rewarding once you start to pay attention. This requires you to slow down and be present so that you don't miss the messages until it's too late and you are laying on the floor in the bathroom. Your body thrives when you take good care of it and it will speak to you when you don't provide it with the right fuel, get enough rest, manage your stress or move enough. Ignoring the messages doesn't make them go away and it certainly doesn't allow for you to feel your best.

Christmas of 2021 was much better for me. Not perfect, but so much better. My day started with overnight oats that I eat every other day of the year, but I still enjoyed one of the muffins. Only one though. I made sure to have a healthy lunch before heading out to visit with family so that I didn't overeat the appetizers. I had a reasonable portion for dinner but will admit that I had a little too much dessert and that sent me over the edge. I didn't feel great after dinner and went home feeling sick to my stomach and lightheaded. Thankfully the feeling passed after about an hour. This was a huge improvement from the previous year where I was a disaster for the entire evening leading into Boxing Day.

We have to learn from these experiences, and determine what we are willing to live with and how we want to feel from the choices we make. There are consequences to how we treat ourselves and having a basis for comparison is helpful. Then we can strive for feeling our best because we know it's worth it. It doesn't mean we won't slip up once in a while, but I know that for me it's a reminder. A strong and forceful one, but a reminder nonetheless. It reminds me of why I eat clean, exercise, get quality sleep, and pay attention to my mental health. If I don't, then I don't feel the way I want to feel and that's good enough for me. That's what continues to drive me forward. Let me point out, though, that part of the reason I still tend to have experiences like Christmas of 2020 is because that relationship I have with food can still be toxic. It still lingers over me, and once in a while, it takes over my better judgment. It continues to be a process for me and I continue to reflect and learn from these experiences in order to better understand myself. This is important work.

I want to feel my best and I want that for you too.

I can only imagine how those that eat like this on a regular basis must feel physically and mentally. The lack of energy, the brain fog, the digestive issues and the list must go on. Yet they don't know any different because they haven't experienced the other side of consistently taking great care of their bodies and feeling amazing inside and out. Again, it doesn't mean you need to be perfect, just consistent. If the norm is having a consistently poor diet, then that's what your body is used to and it's as if it learns to function at that level; even though it's a very low level of functioning. You can do better, though, and you deserve better. You can experience more energy throughout the day. You can clear the brain fog and operate clearly and concisely. You can feel amazing physically and mentally by simply making small adjustments, over time. Don't you want that for yourself?

As I said at the beginning, this book isn't about subscribing to another diet or a book with a step-by-step list of rules for you to follow, only to have you gradually unfollow them. That's not what you need and it's certainly not a good place to start if you want real change this time.

When you start to make changes to your self-care, I want you to think of it like a funnel. You start at the top and continue to narrow in on habits and zero in on things as you experience success, as habits start to become part of who you are and what you do. They become natural because they have been built on a strong foundation, built to consider you and your lifestyle.

You are looking for real change that stems from the inner work and does not involve the diet mentality.

Beyond everything I've already discussed and shared with you, I do feel compelled to provide you with a few additional habits that you can take with you as a starting point. Please know that before you dive in, I want you to take the time to consider all of the inner work topics we've already discussed. That's where you really need to start. If that means you need to go back and reread previous chapters, do it. It's worth it. We have to get our heads on straight before we start putting the other pieces together, otherwise you won't have created the foundation for success. I don't want you feeling overwhelmed and feeling like you have started yet another diet.

These additional habits are ones that you may not have even thought about before or even realized could have a big impact on your success. Either way, you still need consistency, so I want you to consider where you're at in your journey. You're reading this book, which is a fantastic start, but my intention for you is that this is the last time you start again. The last time you start from the beginning.

As stated in chapter one, you don't need to start implementing all of these habits, all at once. In fact, it's better if you don't. One habit at a time, one day at a time. Build that confidence and build on your success.

Be Kind & Patient With Yourself:

This might seem cheesy or obvious, but it needs to be said. You can't move forward with anything else until you recognize that you need to be kind and patient with yourself. This starts your journey off on a positive note and the constant reminder of kindness and patience will allow you to stay in a positive headspace, even when things get tough. You need to allow time and grace while you implement new habits. Nobody else is going to do this for you, so practice this even if it feels uncomfortable.

Start With Areas of Confidence:

As I've said before, you can't just jump in and start everything all at once. You will get overwhelmed and quit before you even get started. So zero in on a couple of areas you feel most confident about and build from there. For example, if drinking more water and going to bed 30 minutes earlier feels manageable to you, start there. If going on a 30 minute walk 3 days a week and increasing the number of vegetables you eat feels like something you can confidently do, start there. Pick 2 or 3 habits to start with and see how you make out. I want you to feel comfortable and confident so that you can create momentum from the successes you gradually achieve.

Recognize Self-Sabotaging Tendencies and Behaviours:

In order to identify when you might be engaging in behaviours that passively or actively go against what it is you are working towards, there needs to be a heightened awareness of your thoughts and actions. You need to pay attention, be present, and take charge of the internal dialogue during those moments. If these behaviours are frequent in nature, there is opportunity for reflection to assess whether you are working towards your goals in a way that actually works for you. There might be room for adjustments to be made to ensure the habits fit with your lifestyle or there may be something bigger at play that requires more specialized attention. Either way, don't let it go and assume the tendencies will simply fade away, as they could be a sign of an unhealthy approach and mindset.

Create a Checklist:

You're more likely to follow through on things if they are written down so I recommend creating a daily checklist. Be sure to include your healthy intentions for the day such as working out, drinking water, planning meals for the following day and anything else you want to be sure to achieve that day. Remember that at the beginning, you are only picking a few habits to start with so the list might be small but it will grow over time. By having them written down, along with anything else you want to accomplish that day, there will be a constant visual reminder for you to reference. There's also the great satisfaction you will get from being able to cross or check off an item from the list!

Pick Movement You Love:

You know that being active is vital and it needs to be one of your non-negotiables, whether you are trying to lose weight or not. You need to move your body and stay strong, and it does wonders for your mental health. I want you to pick a form of movement that you love. Okay, you may not love it, but you enjoy it and can imagine yourself doing it on a consistent basis. The options are endless, so there has to be something you can find and stick with, at least for now as you are starting out. You don't have to commit to an hour a day, just long enough that you feel you've pushed yourself and stepped outside of your comfort zone, even a little. Remember this is just a starting point.

Sleep is a Must:

We've all been told since we were babies how important sleep is, and that doesn't change when we become adults. Having a healthy bedtime routine and getting quality sleep for seven to nine hours creates a solid foundation for many of the other healthy habits you will work on over time. You know how good you feel when you've had a good night's sleep and the impact it has on your energy and ability to be productive and make good choices. Unfortunately, it's one of those areas we don't give too much thought to as we simply go to bed, wake up and move on with our day. I want you to give some thought to what you do before bed, the time you go to bed, your sleep conditions and surroundings, how and when you wake up, and where you might be able to make some improvements. I want you to wake up on the right side of the bed feeling your best each and every day!

Physical AND Mental Satisfaction From Food:

Gaining both physical and mental satisfaction from food is an area I feel is often overlooked. It seems as though the idea of eating healthy means our food will be boring and unsatisfying, both mentally and physically. We have been conditioned to think that if we remove processed foods and sugar, we will be left feeling empty and deprived. This is why it's important to consider not only the physical satisfaction you get from your food, but the mental satisfaction. The taste, flavour, smell, texture and overall sensation of your taste buds. It might sound ridiculous, but it's important. You could eat a plain piece of chicken, some plain brown rice and broccoli, and feel physically satisfied by this meal; but if you were to analyze how mentally satisfied you feel by this meal, it would likely fall short. The result? While you have already consumed enough calories from your meal, you will crave something else and that something else likely won't be healthy. This is where the deprivation comes in and the potential for overeating. When planning and preparing your meals, be sure to consider mental satisfaction. You should look forward to it and while eating it, you should gain a level of enjoyment from it. Yes, it's absolutely possible to eat healthy and love your meals!

Protein, Carbs & Healthy Fats:

The idea of what goes into our meals to make them healthy is the baseline for all diets, which is why I'm not going to lecture you on what you should eat and what you shouldn't eat. It's not as cut and dry as that if we want long-lasting healthy nutrition habits. If we were to simply look at the three primary macronutrients that we would like to consistently make up your meals and snacks, they would be proteins, carbohydrates (fibre) and healthy fats. Ideally you want all three to be included in each of your meals to create balance. This is all I want you to focus on when you start to pay attention to the food you put in your body. We just want awareness to start out. Not perfection. If this concept can be on your radar on a daily basis, you will begin to create meals that are more balanced and definitely more physically and mentally satisfying. You might be asking what are the healthy sources of proteins, carbohydrates and healthy fats you could incorporate into your day, so I decided to make a small list for each, so you have a jumping off point.

> Protein: chicken, turkey, lean beef, lean pork, shellfish, seafood, white fish, salmon, beans, lentils, plain Greek yogurt, eggs, tempeh, tofu

> Carbohydrates: whole grain oats, brown/black/wild rice, quinoa, whole grain breads/wraps, fruits, vegetables, potatoes and sweet potatoes, barley, corn, whole grain pasta

> Healthy Fats: avocado, extra virgin olive oil, avocado oil, olives, nut butters, nuts and seeds such as almonds, walnuts, pumpkin seeds, chia seeds and ground flax.

These lists, by no means, represent a complete picture of healthy food options. Remember, I'm not here to tell you exactly what to eat, when to eat and how to eat. I just want you to be aware of the three categories so you can begin to make an effort to incorporate them into your world. When you're ready of course. You can continue to narrow in on cleaner choices as time goes on, but for now I would encourage you to start thinking in terms of proteins, carbohydrates and healthy fats when you prepare your meals and snacks.

Think of the Week as a Whole:

Rather than simply thinking and planning your meals, snacks, workouts, etc., for a given day, I would love for you to start thinking of your entire week as a whole. This allows you to see the big picture when it comes to how you are really making out with your self-care. Generally, you know what life has in store for you for the upcoming week in terms of work, kids' activities, social functions and community activities. Based on these things, you can start to plan meals, schedule workouts, assess your bedtime and wake up times, and so much more. You know that if on Monday and Thursday you won't have time for a workout, you can then plan to get workouts in on Tuesday, Wednesday and Friday. You know that if you have dinner out planned for Saturday where you may choose to indulge in sweets and alcohol, then leading up to Saturday, you have an opportunity to make healthier choices so that your indulgence isn't repeated all week long. By looking at the week as a whole, you are in a much better position to make choices that create balance throughout the week, and you can start to be intentional with your behaviours based on the big picture.

Be Honest With Yourself:

The final thing I really want you to reflect on before making decisions about where you go from here is how honest you are with yourself. Not only right now, but throughout the process of integrating self-care habits into your life. It does nothing but hinder progress when you try to convince yourself of something, or when you're not willing to admit how you are truly feeling and what thoughts you are actually thinking. You can only suppress the truth for so long before it comes bubbling to the surface. This is why you need to start with honesty. Honesty about what you're truly ready, willing and able to do, and honesty around how you are feeling as you move through the process of change. Have conversations with yourself. Honest conversations. If it's too difficult to have them with yourself, write your thoughts down or speak with someone you trust. When I'm working with a client, I'm constantly checking in to make sure we're on the right path and I expect honesty and full disclosure before we move forward with anything or continue on with a specific habit. You need to be upfront with yourself and understand that by continuously being honest with yourself about where you're at, you will be in a better position to implement change and avoid the starting and restarting of habits.

In earlier chapters, there were many concepts and considerations we discussed in great detail that are part of the inner work I feel so strongly needs to be done. I thought it might be helpful to quickly highlight them again so you can easily reference them down the road.

Ready, willing, able – assess your level of each before proceeding with new health habits to determine where to start, and reassess often as your feelings may change.

Do it for yourself – any new habits should be done based on your best interest, not the interest or approval of others.

Custom strategies – when looking to integrate new habits into your daily routine such as exercise, develop strategies that take into consideration your lifestyle, your likes and dislikes, your career and your family so you can move forward in a realistic manner.

Determine your why – there has to be an understanding of what you truly want to achieve and what will be different if you were successful; only then can you place personal meaning and value on new habits.

Trial and error – sometimes it takes a few tries to figure out what and how healthy habits will actually stick before finding your way.

Start small – taking incremental steps towards your goals allows time for confidence and momentum to build and avoids feelings of overwhelm.

Set yourself up for success – aim for favourable outcomes by creating realistic expectations and routines for yourself that allow you to progress and grow in a way that is proactive and planned.

Meal planning – a necessary evil that will provide you with freedom throughout the week. It will remove the guesswork and will help you avoid false expectations about choosing healthy meals and snacks when life gets crazy around you.

Non-negotiables – pick a few simple habits related to exercise, food, sleep or stress management. Honour the commitments you make to these habits and feel empowered by your ability to put these habits first.

Say NO – get comfortable saying it and remember *why* you are saying it.

Setting boundaries – understand what works for you and what doesn't work for you in order to make decisions that continuously serve you and create the lifestyle you want.

Give yourself choices – choices allow you to feel in control with a sense of freedom and avoid the feeling of being boxed in, resulting in feelings of deprivation while begrudging the process.

Unsubscribe to the diet mentality – let go of the preconceived ideas you have been taught around what it takes to lose weight and to get healthy, and instead, focus on you and what will work best for you.

Create your support system – surround yourself with people that understand you, support you and those you can rely on to share challenges and successes.

Discipline vs motivation – don't rely on motivation to keep moving you forward; instead, understand that you must be disciplined with your behaviours and actions, and motivation will grow from that.

Consistency vs perfection - perfect doesn't exist, so step away from thinking you need to be perfect in order to achieve your goals. Focus on consistent demonstration of habits that bring you closer to your goals.

If you are feeling a sense of overwhelm after reviewing the concepts, take a breath and remind yourself that you will go slow. You will only take on what you can handle and will only move forward at a pace that works for you. Remember this time is going to be different. You are taking a new approach that will likely feel uncomfortable, but it's important to recognize that what you've done in the past has not worked. It has not left you feeling healthy, physically or mentally, and that's what you're after.

You are taking your power back and giving yourself a voice again.

Your voice will know what it wants, will go after it and will see you for the amazing individual you are. You deserve to feel strong, confident and powerful in your body and about your body. You need to start relying on yourself to make decisions and choices that you know will work because you know yourself better than anyone else. So it's time you started calling the shots.

If it helps to highlight the concepts with a bright yellow highlighter, then do it. This is your book. Do what it takes to keep the inner work at the forefront of your mind and present in everything you do. It doesn't mean you won't regress a little or doubt yourself a little, but you can always come back to this safe place and remind yourself of where you're going and why.

Anyone can follow a diet. Anyone can sign up for a fitness program. I don't want you to be just anyone because you know it doesn't last. You know it's not the solution. Healing the wounds you have related to body image, weight loss, diets, and how you feel in your own skin doesn't happen overnight. It can be hard and sometimes very painful, especially when you're focusing on the inner work. I want you to keep showing up and doing the work because it matters; it will pay off and will always be worth it.

As I continue to move forward in my own journey following my own unique path, I know there will be obstacles, detours and setbacks, but I'm now confident in myself and trust in myself. You will get there, too. Remember I hear you, feel you and see you.

You're not alone.

Made in the USA
Middletown, DE
07 October 2022